1-DAY-AT-A-TIME DIET

Also by Joe D. Goldstrich, M.D.:

The Best Chance Diet

1-DAY-AT-A-TIME DIET

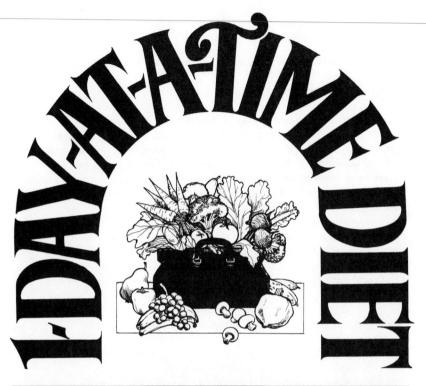

JOE D. GOLDSTRICH, M.D.

with

Daniel Kaufman

Original Recipes by "Mama" Edythe Goldstrich

Foreword by Philip Raskin, M.D.

Knightsbridge Publishing Company
New York

Published in the United States by
Knightsbridge Publishing Company
255 East 49th Street
New York, New York 10017

Library of Congress Cataloging-in-Publication Data

Goldstrich, Joe D.
    1-Day-at-a-Time Diet / by Joe D.
    Goldstrich with Daniel
    Kaufman. — 1st ed.
        p.   cm.
    ISBN 1-877961-14-0 : $18.95
    1. Reducing diets.   2. Nutrition.
3. Health.   4. Reducing diets—
Recipes.   5. Food—Tables.
I. Kaufman, Daniel.   II. Title.
III. Title: 1-Day-at-a-Time Diet
RM222.2.G617   1990
613.2'5—dc20   90-4078
                                CIP

Designed by Mike Yazzolino

Illustrations by Kersti O'Leary

10 9 8 7 6 5 4 3 2
First Edition

For Barbara, my true love

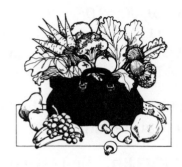

Contents

Lifestyle: Guide to Weight Loss and Health Maintenance   99

The Master Plan: Putting It All Together   151

Recipes   161

Index of Recipes   269

Major changes in your diet may result in major changes in your blood chemistries and may affect medication requirements.

Before beginning any diet, you should consult a physician.

My experience with diabetics taking diabetes medication is that there will be a substantial lowering of the blood sugar on this diet. If you are a diabetic on medication, you will probably require less medicine as a result of this diet. Inform your physician that you are beginning a *low-calorie diet*. Work with your physician in monitoring your changing needs for medication to insure safe and healthy results.

The Jump-Start phase of this diet is not recommended for pregnant and lactating women.

—*The Authors*

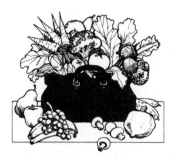

Foreword

Almost everybody I know has tried to lose weight at one time or another. If you are reading this book for that reason, you have a lot of company. Obesity is nearly epidemic in the United States—it is estimated that 25 percent of Americans are overweight. Some of us are just a few pounds heavier than we'd like to be, while others bear the physical and psychological burden of more than a hundred extra pounds. Thus, *1-Day-at-a-Time Diet* has been written at a good time. There are certainly a lot of people who will benefit from Dr. Goldstrich's advice.

Body weight is determined by a relatively simple relationship: the balance between how many calories you take in and how many you burn up during a day. If you consume 3,500 calories more than you expend, you will gain a pound, and if you burn 3,500 calories more than you consume, you will lose a pound. No matter what you may have heard, you cannot defy the laws of thermodynamics! There are, however, differences in the rates at which individuals burn calories. Dr. Goldstrich says he has a "sluggish" metabolism. That means his "equipment" is very fuel-efficient, not unlike an automobile that gets forty miles to a gallon of gas. Other people, the lucky ones, have less efficient motors and only get ten miles to the gallon. Dr. Goldstrich and many of the rest of us need much less fuel to travel the same distance. If you take in more fuel than you need, the human fuel tank expands—and you get fat. There are two ways, then, to reduce your weight: You can decrease your daily calorie input, or you can increase your caloric expenditure through exercise. Dr. Goldstrich's book shows you how to do both.

Joe Goldstrich has been my friend for twenty years. I have always known that he marches to a different drummer, so I am not surprised that he has devised a diet plan that suggests you eat only nonfat yogurt for breakfast, lunch, and dinner on one day, and only potatoes on another. Although these recommendations appear somewhat unorthodox, his book contains much good information and advice. Dr. Goldstrich recommends diets that are low in salt, saturated fat, and cholesterol, and high in complex carbohydrates. This is excellent nutritional advice and is identical to recommendations made by both the American Heart Association and the American Diabetes Association. His book reflects the same loving care he dispenses every day to his patients. Moreover, there are dozens of excellent recipes and many useful tips that will help you avoid the pitfalls of dieting and maintain the "new you."

I hope you enjoy using this innovative book. I wish you success in achieving your weight-loss goal and in continuing to follow the healthy dietary suggestions outlined in 1-Day-at-a-Time Diet.

Philip Raskin, M.D.
University of Texas
Southwestern Medical Center at Dallas

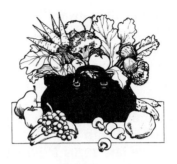

Hungry?

So was I. At age 17 I was 50 pounds overweight. That did not help my social life or my self-esteem at all, so 35 years ago I began reading books on diet and nutrition. I read just about everything that had been written; if it said something about losing weight, I needed to know it. Even though I lost 45 pounds in my first two months of dieting, I always felt (and still feel) the constant threat that the weight might come back unless I took special precautions. I am convinced that 90 percent of all people who have a similar chronic obsession with weight loss are afflicted with a sluggish metabolism, as I am—the kind that shows no mercy toward the minor indulgences and pleasures that we all love so much.

So it's been a lifelong struggle for me, and I've learned over these past 35 years how to make the struggle a little more fun and how to stack the odds in my favor. That's what I'd like to share with you in this book.

As time went on, a number of my relatives died of heart disease, and even though I was maintaining my weight, I became acutely aware of some connection between diet and illness that might occur later. And I heard many warnings about cholesterol. So when I decided to become a physician, I chose as my specialty the field of cardiology, with a subspecialty of arteriosclerosis and its treatment by diet. Later I became the national director of education and community programs for the American Heart Association, and worked with the AHA nutrition program.

In the late 1970s I sought out Nathan Pritikin to learn more about nutrition, weight loss, and heart disease. I became Pritikin's medical confidant. He was a genius who had taught himself medicine, but because he lacked clinical hands-on experience as a physician, he turned to me for advice concerning the clinical application of some of his theories.

My association with Nathan Pritikin had a tremendous benefit for me as well. I learned about his diet directly from the horse's mouth, and I began to eat as Pritikin taught. In a few short months, I lost 15 pounds, and my cholesterol dropped from 210 to 150. I was very pleased with the results, and I thought that my eating woes were over forever. But the Pritikin regimen didn't leave much room for those dietary pleasures that I mentioned above, and after a while I eventually strayed from the path. The same old sluggish metabolism was still there, ready to claim its pounds at the slightest invitation. I had still more to learn.

Having mastered what Pritikin had to teach about diet and nutrition, I moved on to study with other nutritional experts. I studied macrobiotics with Michio Kushi, the founder and world leader of the macrobiotic movement. When a mutual friend introduced us in Dallas, we went to a Japanese restaurant for dinner. Kushi ate enormous quantities of food, bowl after bowl. I was convinced that this man knew something important about diet, nutrition, and weight loss. Despite the huge quantities of food he consumed, his weight remained slim and healthy, like Pritikin's. I read his books, and had the opportunity to study with him personally a few months later.

A year or so after studying with Michio Kushi, I read about Anne Wigmore's raw-foods diet.

I continued to study with as many of the great teachers of nutrition as possible, and I've read most of the books on diet and nutrition that have been written in the last 25 years. I've tried to learn something from each of them. The 1-Day-at-a-Time diet incorporates what I've learned over this quarter of a century in both my studies and in dealing with literally thousands of patients on a nutritional level.

I tend to look for the valid principles underlying various diets and approaches to nutrition. For example, if you look at Anne Wigmore's raw-foods diet and compare it to Michio Kushi's macrobiotic diet, on the surface you might see no similarity. In macrobiotics all of the food is cooked; in the raw-foods diet none of the food is cooked. So if the principle that food must be cooked to make it digestible is true, then the raw-foods diet is invalid. But if the principle that cooking destroys all the natural enzymes in the food, which is espoused by the raw-foods followers, is true, then the macrobiotic diet is totally invalid. In truth, both of these are useful diets for some people at some points in their lives.

Common Principles

What are the common underlying truths in both the macrobiotic and raw-foods diets?

1. Both are *low-fat* diets (there is no added fat in either diet).
2. Both are comprised of *complex carbohydrates*.
3. Both use *unprocessed natural foods*.
4. Both are *free of sugar and refined products*.
5. Both include a lot of *fiber and roughage*.

The macrobiotic principles of Kushi and the raw-foods approach of Wigmore are both in keeping with the Pritikin diet. If you look at other diets that work, you find these same principles: they use whole foods that are unprocessed, that are high in complex carbohydrates and fiber, and that are low in fats and oils. Also, neither of these diets uses eggs; we'll talk more about eggs later.

Why Diet Books Fail

The reason that some diet books fail in their purpose to help you lose weight is this: *You must incorporate the principles of healthy eating into your life on a day-to-day basis* in order to lose weight and maintain weight loss. Any do-it-quick, short-term program is doomed to failure because it doesn't teach you the information you need to know to lose weight on a long-term basis.

That's why Weight Watchers is so effective; they teach you to lose weight in a healthy way over the long haul. You can't expect short-term solutions to long-term problems. The solution to the problem of weight requires a re-education. It requires a *long-term commitment* to your own health and well-being.

The 1-Day-at-a-Time Diet

The time has come for the 1-Day-at-a-Time diet; it is a simple, exciting, and effective eating plan that not only delivers immediate weight loss but also teaches you the principles of a lifelong, healthy dietary lifestyle.

Half a Pound of Weight Loss per Day

I recommend that everyone who goes on the 1-Day-at-a-Time diet get themselves a good scale. Ordinary bathroom scales are not adequate because they don't have reproducible, consistent weights. You can purchase a decent digital scale for about $35. The benefit of this is that if you weigh yourself each day, you get instantaneous feedback about what you've accomplished the previous day, and you'll know that you're continuing to make progress.

Now, remember that when you begin this diet, your initial weight loss (mostly water loss) will be great. It's not unreasonable to expect to see two to four pounds lost on the first day with the 1-Day-at-a-Time diet. But as time goes on and this bloat of excess water is lost, the rate of weight loss will not be as great. What would you like to lose on a long-term basis? In the beginning weeks it is totally realistic to expect *half a pound of weight loss per day* if you follow the principles detailed in this book, without counting calories, but simply staying with this effortless, proven program.

What does half a pound of weight loss per day mean? It means a great deal: It means *15 pounds a month*! It also means 170 pounds a year, although that's too much to really expect unless you weigh over 400 pounds.

In my diet seminars, the lowest weight loss was 4 pounds in one week, and the highest was 17 pounds.

Eating one food per day improves the digestion and the metabolism; the body becomes a more efficient machine. So don't be surprised if you see gains even greater than those stated here. And if you follow the Lifestyle principles (see page 103) you will experience dramatic improvements in other areas of your health as well.

POTENTIAL BENEFITS OF THE 1-DAY-AT-A-TIME DIET

- Eliminates the boredom of dieting
- Makes possible lasting weight loss without counting calories
- Improves the cardiovascular system
- Strengthens the immune system
- Slows down the aging process
- Increases self-esteem through self-control

- Teaches you all of the basic principles of healthful eating
- Gives you the potential to lose a half pound per day
- Eliminates constipation
- Balances blood sugar
- Lowers cholesterol in the blood
- Lowers blood pressure
- Raises vitality and energy level

The 1-Day-at-a-Time Diet

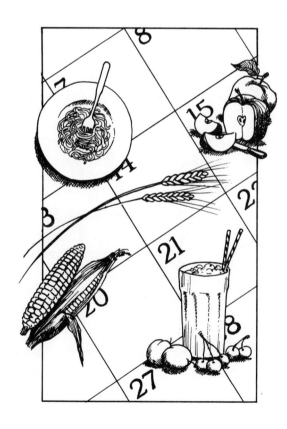

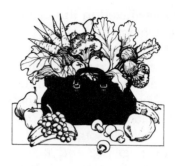

The 1-Day-at-a-Time diet is in two parts: The first section, Jump-Start, will provide weight loss in the *short* run, and will also *educate* you about certain healthy foods. The second section, Lifestyle, will produce weight loss over the long run, and will show you exactly how to *maintain* a steady weight loss and good health.

Jump-Start

This phase of the 1-Day-at-a-Time diet lets you manage your food consumption *one day at a time*. There are certain foods that can be eaten in large quantities, and not only will they satisfy your hunger, they will also help you to lose weight. These very special foods can be eaten almost without limitation—that is, *you can even eat all you want of some of these foods, satisfy your hunger, and still lose weight!*

The one-a-day foods in Jump-Start are really the building blocks of the Lifestyle phase "maintenance diet." These foods are intermixed in the maintenance diet, which is actually an extension of the mix and match days of Jump-Start. The foods introduced in Jump-Start, the foods that you eat exclusively for a day at a time, are exactly the same foods that will be eaten together in the Lifestyle phase of this diet.

In Jump-Start, I will show you step by step how to eat certain foods, one food a day, and in two cases—vegetables and vegetable soup (see Edythe's Fresh Vegetable Soup recipe on pages 62 and 196)—as much as you want of that food. I'll also tell you what foods to eat each day so that your energy and your appetite will be balanced to enable you to lose the maximum amount of weight.

Although I've outlined a very specific plan for Jump-Start (see page 23), it's not cast in concrete. Some people will love the vegetables but find that eating twelve pieces of fruit a day makes them a little gassy. Others will love the fruit but find that the vegetables make them gassy. *Be flexible!* If a specific day does not agree with you, convert it to a Mix and Match Day, using the foods and principles described in How to Use This Diet (see page 15). If you need more flexibility, refer to How to Chart Your Own Jump-Start (see page 21), and read Mix and Match Day (page 85).

If you use only the Mix and Match days for all of Jump-Start, your weight loss will still be significant and you will have learned the important principles of the 1-Day-at-a-Time diet. If you find that one food a day is not for you, go to the Lifestyle phase (see page 99) and use the menu outlined in the Master Plan (see page 156). If you use only the Master Plan—surprise! Your weight loss will still be significant. *There's something for everyone in this book!*

Jump-Start will give you the best of short-term weight loss and at the same time start you on a process for long-term revamping of your eating style. I've used these tricks over the years, and I know it is relatively easy to lose *five to seven pounds in one week* and still maintain a high level of energy.

Much of the initial weight loss in Jump-Start is bloat

that comes from too much salt and fats in the diet. The reason for this is that fats influence the circulation in such a way that makes it more difficult for the kidneys to eliminate salt and water, which is therefore retained as bloat. So when you lose five to seven pounds in one week, it doesn't mean that you've lost five to seven pounds of fatty tissue. But you can get rid of the excess weight in salt and water that your body is carrying around, and at the same time improve your circulation and enhance the performance of your kidneys, liver, and other vital organs. You have to realize that when you drop the five to seven pounds, there is then a restabilization period, and this is the most crucial time of all; if you go back to eating the way you did before, you'll put the five to seven pounds back on just as easily as you originally gained them, and you'll get nowhere. Besides, the up-and-down see-saw is a real strain on the body.

In the Jump-Start phase of the 1-Day-at-a-Time diet, you eat only one type of food each day. Sometimes you can even eat all you want of that one food. *You don't need a computer to keep track of calories or foods if you do your dieting one-day-at-a-time!*

In fact, one common statement about Jump-Start I hear from my diet seminar participants is: "We hated the kinds of diets where you had to measure every little thing and always had to be thinking about preparing the next meal. What we really like about this diet is that it is so simple. It's real easy and you don't have to think a lot about it, you can just do it."

What happens is that the more you eat of that one food, the more satiated you become, and the more likely you are to lose your appetite. Even though you can have plenty of that particular food, your desire for more will diminish. In addition, eating one food a day, in my experience, leads to *increased efficiency* in digestion so that the body can burn that one food easier and weight loss is facilitated.

By eating just one food a day, you also eliminate the

most common source of failure in diet: *the loss of willpower*. When you're on a diet and you're not committed to eating just one particular food a day, you go to the refrigerator or into the pantry and look for something to eat because you're still hungry. Then you say, "No, I don't want this; no, I don't want that," and you end up eating something that's not healthy.

With this phase of the 1-Day-at-a-Time diet you don't have these choices to make. All you have to do is to make your commitment each day to eating *just that one food* for the day. Then there is no question, "Am I going to eat this chocolate bar; am I going to eat that piece of pie?" You've made your commitment *one-day-at-a-time* to eat only vegetables, to eat only fruits, or pasta, rice, or soup, or whatever you choose from the list.

This diet works because once you know you can have more brown rice or more squash or more of that one food, then the decisions are all made for you. That's half the battle. You just make the commitment that today you're going to adhere to the plan.

Another advantage of Jump-Start is that no matter how bored or unhappy you are with one food, tomorrow is a new day, tomorrow's another experience. If it was brown rice today, tomorrow it can be frozen yogurt, or fruit—you always have something to look forward to.

There's been a lot written recently about food combining. The Jump-Start phase of the 1-Day-at-a-Time diet is the ultimate food combination! There is no worry about food combining because you're only combining with the same thing, which is a perfect combination every time. You don't have to worry about digestion. Rice goes perfectly with rice, rice and fruit go well together, and rice and vegetables mix well together. I'll tell you more about the mix and match principles later on.

Jump-Start is a technique you can use one day a week, or seven days a week. Use it to achieve short-term goals (like getting into that new dress or bathing suit). Or use it to initiate a longer-term weight-loss program. You can follow Jump-Start for a week or two before going on to the maintenance program (Lifestyle, see page 99). If weight loss slows on the maintenance program you can always return to Jump-Start. Over the long haul it is the maintenance part of this program, Lifestyle, that will insure your good health and slimness.

Lifestyle

Fifty million Americans are obese or overweight. Our most common diseases are all linked to the typical American diet. It is now understood how most degenerative diseases result from an unhealthy lifestyle. Understanding the basic nutrition principles detailed in this book and *following these guidelines* in your daily life will eliminate most if not all of the diseases associated with poor diet. There is a massive amount of evidence, both from government and private studies, supporting all of the principles of the Lifestyle phase in this book. As one of my diet seminar participants noted about Lifestyle: "What you have done for me is gotten me to think about what I eat. I used to eat nuts, cheese, things that I shouldn't eat. You have educated my mind and now I think about what I eat."

Even if you do not wish to stay with the Jump-Start phase of the 1-Day-at-a-Time diet, you can go on to the Lifestyle phase and still enjoy all of the weight loss and health benefits of the 1-Day-at-a-Time diet. The Lifestyle phase is the maintenance part of this diet, and you won't have to count calories or deprive yourself of variety if you just *follow the menu and lifestyle principles* detailed in this phase.

If you do choose to try out the Jump-Start phase for an impressive short-term weight loss, you must realize that to maintain your weight loss and your good health you must incorporate the advice given in the Lifestyle phase. I have been doing nutritional counseling in my medical practice for over 10 years and have prescribed diets for literally thousands of people. The basic principles of proper diet remain essentially the same for everyone:

- Eliminate excess fats and oils.
- Eat complex carbohydrates.
- Emphasize vegetables and fruits.
- Stay away from sugars and processed foods.

If you do all this, you're going to become slim and healthy, and you're going to stay that way for the rest of your life.

How to Use
This Diet

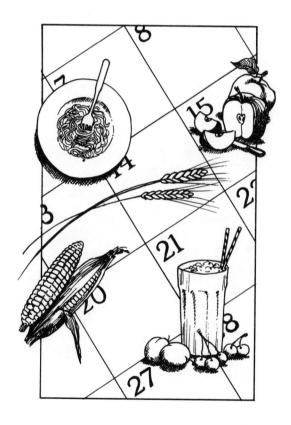

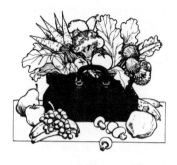

In the Jump-Start phase of the 1-Day-at-a-Time diet, I introduce you to several foods that you can eat by themselves all day long. These are exactly the same foods that will form the building blocks of the Lifestyle phase, or maintenance portion of the diet. I give you 13 different options during Jump-Start, including a Mix and Match Day and a day in which you repeat your favorite food from the 11 one-day-at-a-time choices.

Go through Jump-Start doing as many of the days as you can. If you get to the middle of a day and you find that it is a real struggle for you, convert that day to a Mix and Match Day (see page 85). One person's favorite day may be someone else's *least* favorite day. I have seen people who have begged to repeat the Fruit Day three or four days in a row because they found it so appealing and so easy to stay with, and others who have had trouble finishing even one Fruit Day because it didn't agree with their system. Each of us is a biochemically unique individual. It is important to respect our own uniqueness and only eat those foods that best match our own individual nature.

The Jump-Start days follow a special order, which may not be initially apparent. They alternate between what I call *light days* and *heavy days*. The Rice, Pasta, Corn, Potato, and Protein Days are the heavy days; the Vegetable, Soup, Fruit, Juice, Frozen Yogurt, and Liquid Protein Days are considered light days. The way I've laid it out, you alternate light and heavy days in order to balance your system. If you ate several light days in a row, your weight loss might initially be faster but you would run the risk of having temporarily low energy or "diet fatigue"; also, the healthy vegetable protein that comes from the grains would be lacking.

If you eat only the heavy days such as the Rice, Corn, Pasta, Potato, and Protein Days, you won't lose weight as fast and you won't learn about the foods that are truly lowest in calorie density. These "low density" foods are the most useful in the Lifestyle phase of this diet for continuing your weight loss and maintaining the benefits that you already have made.

The length of time spent on Jump-Start will vary from person to person. My experience in prescribing this diet to my patients has been that if you use the first seven days as I have outlined them for you, you will lose somewhere between four and seven pounds, depending on how much initial weight you have to lose. You may elect to utilize Jump-Start for a full 13 days, or you may be ready for other options after the first week. I recommend that you *do not use Jump-Start for more than 13 days in a row.*

When you are ready to move on from Jump-Start, here are your options:

Option 1. Go directly to Lifestyle (see page 99) and begin using the Lifestyle phase menu (see the Master Plan Menu, page 156).

Option 2. Use the Lifestyle phase menu three or four

days a week and then use three or four of your favorite "one-day-at-a-times" from Jump-Start the rest of the week. You may choose to alternate Lifestyle and Jump-Start days.

Option 3. Go on the Lifestyle diet for a week or two; stabilize your weight loss, and you will probably lose several more pounds in the process. Then return to Jump-Start for another week to maximize your weight loss once again. Then begin the cycle all over again, depending on how much more weight you want to lose. Eventually you will be on Lifestyle for the rest of your life in order to maintain and/or continue your weight loss.

My experience with people who use Lifestyle exclusively is that their weight loss averages between one and four pounds a week, depending on how much weight they have to lose.

If you stray from the path and have a day when you blow your diet, simply return to one of the light days of Jump-Start and you will be able to rapidly undo all of the damage you did. When you step off the path it only means that it is time to step back on the path. You will not wreck the progress that you have worked so hard to accomplish. Just get back on it the next day.

People have written about the benefits of fasting, where they consume nothing but water or juice for days or even weeks in a row. I don't believe this is a healthy way to eat, because it creates an imbalance in the system. Extending Jump-Start and eating only one food a day could, after many weeks, also cause an imbalance in your system. For this reason I recommend that you not use the pure Jump-Start phase for longer than 13 days in a row. This will keep your system in balance.

Water and Other Beverages

Unlike on other diets, it's not necessary to drink extra liquids on the 1-Day-at-a-Time diet. The foods that make up this diet are all rich in water instead of calories. Most people report an increase in urination on this diet without additional intake of liquids.

A lot of diet and health practitioners make a general statement about how much liquid a person should drink each day. I've never found the perfect formula that fits every person. Fortunately, our bodies are endowed with an exquisite mechanism for regulating fluid balance: when we need more water, we get thirsty. It's important to listen to your body and drink water when your body tells you to. I've never seen anyone get into trouble by doing this.

Water. The healthiest thing to drink is water. I prefer purified or bottled water whenever possible.

Diet drinks, coffee, and tea. Many people are addicted to caffeine. It's not uncommon for people to drink four or more caffeinated beverages a day, such as soft drinks, coffee, and tea. Too much caffeine is not healthy, and we should all work toward reducing and eventually eliminating caffeine from our diet.

The artificial sweetener used in most diet sodas, Nutrisweet, serves no useful purpose within the body, and its intake should be limited. If you must drink diet sodas, hold it to two per day maximum.

Alcohol. Alcohol is a controversial subject. It's a major source of hidden calories for many people. You'll do much better if you eliminate alcohol entirely during Jump-Start and limit your intake to no more than two drinks (glasses of wine, light beer, or cocktail) per day in the Lifestyle phase.

The 1-Day-at-a-Time Recipes

You can use the recipes that are included in the individual Jump-Start days to add variety to your meals. All of the recipes in Jump-Start may also be used in the Lifestyle phase of the 1-Day-at-a-Time diet. These recipes are all low in fat, high in complex carbohydrates, and full of healthy nutrition that will support your lifelong Lifestyle eating habits.

We have not included the specific nutritional breakdown of each recipe, because it's not necessary. If you only put healthy ingredients into the recipe, the final product will always be healthy: low in fat and low in calories.

How to Chart Your Own Jump-Start

I recommend that you follow the order of Jump-Start as it's presented in this book. However, if you want to make changes or alter the order, follow these guidelines:

- Always begin Day 1 with Rice Day.
- Follow Rice Day with a "light" day (vegetables, soup, fruit, juice, yogurt, liquid protein).
- Alternate "light" and "heavy" (pasta, corn, rice, potato, protein) days.
- Choose from eleven 1-day-at-a-time foods (rice, vegetables, pasta, fruit, potatoes, soup, protein, yogurt, corn, juice, liquid protein); add a Mix and Match Day; repeat your favorite day.
- Be flexible. If you start a day and it's not working for you, convert it to a Mix and Match Day. Remember to follow the basic Lifestyle principles listed below.
- Do not stay on Jump-Start for more than 13 days in a row. At the end of 13 days, go to the Lifestyle phase (see page 99) for a week or two; then, if necessary, return to Jump-Start for further maximum weight loss.
- Take it one day at a time! Tomorrow is a new day!

LIFESTYLE PRINCIPLES

- Eliminate excess fats and oils.
- Eat complex carbohydrates (rice, grains, pasta, potatoes).
- Emphasize vegetables and fruits.

- Stay away from sugars and processed foods.
- Exercise!
- Eat moderate amounts of protein.
- Consume only nonfat dairy products.
- Use salt with caution.
- Don't forget fiber!
- Start the day right with breakfast.
- Eat less and live longer!
- Supplement your diet with vitamins and minerals.
- Snack wisely.
- Make intelligent decisions in restaurants.
- Use your mind to help heal your body.

SHOPPING LIST TO BEGIN THE 1-DAY-AT-A-TIME DIET

1. One to two pounds of brown rice
2. Lots of your favorite vegetables for Vegetable Day and plenty of extra vegetables for snacking and for Soup Day
3. Twelve ounces of spaghetti or pasta noodles, and no-oil pasta sauce or ingredients to make your own pasta sauce (see Marinara Sauce recipe, pages 46 and 227)
4. Twelve pieces of fruit for Fruit Day
5. Eight russet baking potatoes
6. Chicken breasts or fish
7. Eight to twelve ears of corn
8. Three quarts of juice (see How Much Juice to Drink, page 83)
9. 1 can of Slim-Fast, or other liquid-protein formula (see page 95)
10. Vitamins (see Vitamin Supplementation, page 143, and The Master Plan, page 151)
11. A dozen eggs for egg-white omelettes or hard-boiled egg whites (see pages 65 and 66)

Jump-Start

The 1-Day-at-a-Time Foods

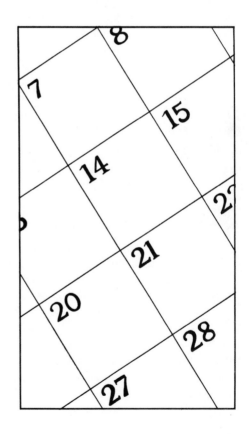

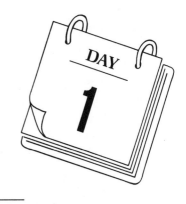

RICE DAY

The Jump-Start phase of the 1-Day-at-a-Time diet should always begin with a day of eating only brown rice. Brown rice is as close to a perfect food as any food can be. The outer hull, which is removed in white rice, contains the B vitamins and is also a rich source of fiber; therefore brown rice is *always* preferable to white rice. In a pinch, however, white rice can be substituted; I'll tell you more about that later.

Not only does brown rice provide a good source of vitamins, minerals, and fabulous fiber, it is also an excellent source of protein and is one of the best complex carbohydrates. Rice provides constant, unfluctuating, and high-power energy fuel for our body engines. Brown rice is a balanced food that facilitates the purification process.

Rice is the staple food of nearly one-half of the world's population. Rice, with its eight essential amino acids, facilitates the cells' efficient use of protein. The form of protein contained in rice is easily assimilated by the body and does not promote coronary artery disease. Rice does not put any strain on the kidneys. It contains almost no fat, and the fat that is present is quite healthy. Rice is truly a miracle food, which is why I urge you to begin your 1-Day-at-a-Time diet with a day of eating only brown rice.

Unless you suffer from low blood pressure, I suggest that you do not use salt or soy sauce in the preparation or eating of brown rice. By eliminating salt you will further aid your body in ridding itself of bloat. If you do have a problem with bloating, it is absolutely essential that you do not use salt during this phase of the diet, and probably later on as well. I'll tell you how to season the rice shortly.

Type of Rice to Use

As long as it's *brown rice*, it does not make any difference whether it is short-grain or long-grain. I have found a gourmet brown rice now available in health-food stores, made by the Lundberg Company. I buy a regular two-pound bag of brown rice, and then add 8 or 12 ounces of the gourmet rice to that. This gives the rice a little special flavor. Wild rice can also be mixed with the brown rice for a delicious variation in flavor and texture.

I tend to rotate; I'll cook up a batch of long-grain rice, and then switch to short-grain the next time. I prefer to use organic rice, which is available in health-food stores, as opposed to the regular brown rice available in grocery stores. The reason for this is that the regular rice has been grown with pesticides, which wouldn't make much difference if you were going to eat just one small serving of rice with the rest of a meal. However, since you will be eating large quantities of rice, it's probably safer not to be putting these chemicals into your body.

Brown Basmati rice is another variation on the theme, and it gives a slightly aromatic, quite pleasant, flavor to the rice.

Cooking the Brown Rice

I've been amazed at how many excellent cooks don't know how to prepare brown rice properly. It's very simple once you get the hang of it. I like to wash the rice first, rinsing it two or three times. You'll see a cloudy substance along with some of the pieces of rice that will float to the surface. Drain the rice, and add twice as much water as you have rice. (If you have two cups of brown rice, for example, add four cups of water.) Put it on the stove and bring it to a boil. Once it reaches boiling point, put a lid on the pot and lower the heat as much as possible. Set a timer for one hour, and leave the rice cooking for the *full hour*. Do not lift the lid to see how the rice is doing; if you lift the lid you lose the head of steam and may spoil the rice. When the hour's up, turn off the heat and with the lid still on the rice, let it sit for another 15 minutes. This seems to improve the flavor.

Seasoning the Rice

Since we're not going to be using salt, how can we give the rice a little additional flavor? I personally prepare my rice without seasoning, which takes a little getting used to. But once you do get used to it, you'll enjoy the wholesome, satisfying rice flavor.

However, if you desire a little variety in the taste of the rice, there are a number of seasonings you can use. There is usually a section of salt-free seasonings in health-food stores and in some regular grocery stores. One company makes a line of seasonings called Instead of Salt; one is for chicken, another for hamburger, one for fish, and one for vegetables. Any one of these can be used as a seasoning for the rice. You can rotate them and have different seasoning at different times. They are all salt-free and contain good herbs. The Mrs. Dash line of salt-free seasonings is also delicious. Vegit is another tasty salt-free seasoning available in health-food stores. Or try making your own (see Seasoning Shaker recipes, pages 187–188). You can also use your own combinations of fresh herbs, such as tarragon or basil.

Another trick is to take some chicken parts—such as legs, wings, and necks—and boil them in 2 quarts of water for an hour and a half or so. At the end of that period take the chicken out and let the broth cool (you will end up with about 1 quart). Refrigerate the broth overnight; the next morning scrape the fat off. You can then use this fat-free chicken broth as the liquid to cook your rice in; it gives the rice a wonderful, rich chicken flavor. You can also pour the chicken stock into an ice tray and put the ice tray in the freezer. When you cook the rice, add a couple of these chicken-broth ice cubes to the water (see Seasoned Chicken Broth and Oriental Chicken Stock recipes, pages 189 and 190).

How Much Rice Can You Eat in a Day?

You don't see many overweight Orientals. They eat essentially unlimited quantities of rice every day, just as Michio Kushi did, and they never seem to gain weight. Rice is a wonderful diet food!

On Rice Day you can eat up to two cups of uncooked rice. Two cups doesn't sound like very much, but that's *uncooked*; two cups of uncooked rice will make about *six* cups of cooked rice, and that's a lot of rice to eat in one day. That should fill up most anyone.

You should spread the six cups of cooked rice out over the entire day; try eating one cup of rice six times a day (one cup at breakfast, a cup between breakfast and lunch, a cup for lunch, a cup in midafternoon, a cup for supper, and a sixth cup between supper and bedtime). Or you could "graze" on smaller amounts of rice all day long to help you lose weight.

How to Prepare for Rice Day

I suggest that you make up your brown rice the day before. It does take an hour of cooking plus another 15 minutes of sitting with the heat off, and you may not have time to do this cooking in the morning. If you make it the night before, you can let it cool overnight outside the refrigerator. It won't spoil. Then the easiest way to heat it up in the morning is to use a double-broiler-type vegetable steamer. Steam the rice until it's hot, which will take only a few minutes. It can also be reheated quickly in a microwave, which is something you can do when you take your rice to work or take it with you elsewhere during the day. You can even reheat your rice in a microwave at any 7-Eleven store.

I recommend that you get some containers to hold approximately one cup of rice at a time. Then after you have your morning rice, you can pack three more cups to take with you to eat during the day. That leaves another cup for dinner and a sixth cup for between dinnertime and bedtime.

White Rice in a Pinch

Although I strongly recommend that you use only brown rice, if you have no facilities to prepare the rice, or if you forget your rice on a Rice Day or whatever, you can always go to an Oriental restaurant and use the plain steamed white rice that they serve. It's not as good—it doesn't have the vitamins or the fiber—but it will provide the energy and it will work essentially the same way as far as this diet is concerned.

Mix and Match with Rice

If you get bored with the rice toward dinnertime and feel that you must have something additional to eat, the best foods to mix with rice are fish, vegetables, or fruit. So if you've been eating brown rice all day and don't want to see another grain of it, you could safely and healthfully have a meal of steamed vegetables for dinner, or two pieces of fruit, or you could have a piece of broiled, poached, or steamed fish. Corn will also combine well with the brown rice.

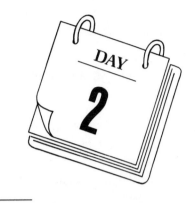

VEGETABLE DAY

I once heard comedian Buddy Hackett tell Johnny Carson that celery had "minus two" calories. When Carson inquired how that could be, Hackett explained that the celery stalk itself has five calories but it takes seven calories of energy to chew and digest it. So the net effect is that celery has minus-two calories, or that you lose weight when you eat celery. This is true to a large extent and is one of the blessings of all vegetables: the water and fiber content is so high that in order to digest vegetables, you use up calories. Vegetable Day is one of the most important days on the 1-Day-at-a-Time diet. It is a day you can come back to time and time again, and it will always benefit your health and your weight-reduction program. There is no limit to the amount of vegetables you can eat on vegetable day.

A Little Protein on Vegetable Day: Egg-Whites

Since, as you will see in the Protein Day section, we're going to let you have a few vegetables on Protein Day (see pages 67–68), it seems only fitting that you could have a little protein on Vegetable Day. So for those of you who aren't quite ready to try cooked vegetables for breakfast, why not have an egg-white omelette or hard-boiled egg whites using as many egg whites as you wish (see Protein Day, pages 65 and 66). The egg-white omelette may contain some sautéed vegetables.

If you prefer to be a real purist, simply start the day with some vegetables. I use frozen vegetables and just put them in the microwave. Choose unsalted frozen vegetables—string beans, okra, broccoli, cauliflower, or combinations of any of those, or squash with carrots and onion, or whatever you like. You can cook them quickly in the microwave, and they taste delicious. You can eat all the cooked vegetables you want for breakfast. Eating vegetables for breakfast is a great weight-reduction maneuver. The water content of the vegetables is so high that the more vegetables you eat, the more weight you are going to lose. Water doesn't have any calories; it is easily lost and will help cleanse your system. If you prefer to eat cooked vegetables and have an egg-white omelette on the side, that is perfectly all right too.

Snacking on Vegetable Day

After breakfast, if you get hungry during the morning, you should eat raw vegetables. It could be raw carrot sticks or celery sticks; or slices of raw cucumber, zucchini, or yellow squash; or a raw tomato. (You wise guys who know that tomatoes are a fruit, don't panic. We are going to allow tomatoes on Vegetable Day, and on Fruit Day too if you like!)

Lunch on Vegetable Day

For lunch on Vegetable Day you have several options. You can once again have cooked vegetables or some raw vegetables.

For Vegetable Day, I keep frozen vegetables in the freezer of my office refrigerator. I have found that Pictsweet makes individual one-serving packs, with a wide variety of vegetables and vegetable combinations. They have a broccoli and cauliflower combination; a zucchini, red pepper, and onion combination; and a corn, tomato, and squash combination. I usually eat two of these packages for a quite filling and satisfying meal. You could also get a large package of frozen vegetables and spoon out as much as you want for your noon meal. Those of you who have the resources and the time and the desire, feel free to prepare fresh vegetables. This can be anything you want—zucchini, onion, and tomato make an excellent combination—and the best way to cook these vegetables is by steaming. Or you could make a vegetable stir-fry in a wok with a couple of chicken-broth ice cubes. For seasonings, try some of the same seasonings mentioned in the Rice Day chapter (see pages 27–28), or try one of the imitation butter sprinkles mentioned in the Potato Day chapter (see page 54).

For those of you who would prefer to have raw vegetables for lunch, the best way to do that is with a salad. You can have as big a salad as you wish. You can even have a huge salad *in addition* to your cooked vegetables.

Eat More Vegetables—Lose More Weight

When I first joined Nathan Pritikin in Santa Barbara in 1977, a famous television personality had recently spent 30 days at the clinic and had gone back to Los Angeles to resume his television duties. However, he continued to eat large salads for lunch and before dinner and continued to lose weight. After a few months his producers sent him back to Pritikin to find out how he could *stop losing weight*; it seems he was no longer so attractive on television because he had gotten too skinny! Pritikin advised him to stop eating salads to curtail his weight loss. I have never forgotten this lesson that I learned from Nathan Pritikin early on: *The more vegetables you eat, the more weight you lose.*

So a huge salad with vegetables for lunch is an excellent choice. You can have all the lettuce you want, and any vegetable you want—tomato, cucumber, radish, green pepper, zucchini—with one exception: avocado. Avocado (actually a fruit) is very fatty and high in calories. After you have lost all the weight you want, it is fine to garnish your salads with a little bit of avocado if you wish, but in this serious weight-reduction mode it is best to avoid avocado. Eat a huge salad, and for those of you who feel you need a little protein at lunch, you can have the white of one or more hard-boiled eggs (but not the yolk) chopped on top of your salad. Even though corn is a vegetable, it is higher in calories than many other vegetables, and therefore is considered as a vegetable for a heavy day. So hold off on eating corn until Corn Day. Beans and peas are even more caloric, and for this reason are not included during Jump-Start.

Acceptable Salad Dressings

At this point we must deal with the important issue of salad dressing. There is a whole spectrum of salad dressings available on the market. Some have as low as 2 to 3 calories per serving and some are as high as 120 or more calories per serving. If you use these high-calorie dressings there will be more calories in the dressing than in the salad itself. This is not a good idea. The lower the calorie content of your salad dressing, the more weight you will lose.

The lowest-calorie dressings include plain lemon juice,

plain vinegar, a combination of lemon juice and vinegar, and some of the commercially available diet salad dressings made without oil. Some of these are quite tasty. Oil is what gives salad dressing its calories, so the no-oil dressings are always going to be lower in calories. I encourage you to experiment with no-oil dressings such as the Pritikin and Estee lines. The Estee products include Thousand Island, blue cheese, creamy cucumber, and a variety of other no-oil dressings. They do, however, have the disadvantage of containing chemical additives and artificial sweetener. Kraft and other companies offer a variety of reduced-calorie dressings. Some have no oil, and some have minimal oil. It's best to use dressings with less than 16 calories per serving. Weight Watchers and Richard Simmons also offer excellent low-calorie, low- or no-oil dressings.

Several of the fast-food restaurants now feature salad bars. Some, such as Wendy's, include a reduced-calorie dressing at their salad bar.

A Word of Caution about Broccoli and Cauliflower

Now that you have had a wonderful all-vegetable lunch, you can have all the raw vegetables you want as a snack between lunch and dinnertime, just as you did in the morning. A word of caution is in order; I learned this the hard way. If you eat raw broccoli and raw cauliflower you're going to experience a lot of gas. So save the broccoli and cauliflower for cooking and concentrate more on things like cucumber, zucchini, carrot, and celery for the raw vegetables.

Dinner on Vegetable Day

For dinner on Vegetable Day, start with a big raw-vegetable salad as the first course. Eat as much of the salad as you like. The second course will be cooked vegetables—what a surprise on Vegetable Day! The vegetables should be steamed; if you have time, they should be fresh. You can steam zucchini with yellow squash, onion, and tomato; you can steam string beans and okra. Many people dislike okra because of its slimy consistency, but it's a low-calorie, high-fiber vegetable that is very beneficial. You can steam broccoli and cauliflower, or cabbage, or Brussels sprouts, or asparagus. Cook about a third more vegetables than you think you will want for the meal. Eat the leftovers cold as your snack later on in the evening if you get hungry. You can actually do this every day during the Lifestyle phase because cooked vegetables should be a part of your evening meal every single day. The vegetables will digest quickly and you will find that your sleep will not be disturbed as it might be if you ate heavier things between dinner and bedtime.

Another Protein Option on Vegetable Day

For those of you who feel that Vegetable Day just does not provide enough protein, one of the ideas you will see in the Mix and Match section is to add a little bit of protein at dinnertime. The best way is with a piece of broiled fish. Another option: a broiled, defatted, skinned chicken breast along with your salad and cooked vegetables. A little reminder here: As a variation on steamed vegetables, you can stir-fry them with *small amounts* of olive oil or stir-fry them in chicken broth. If you've made up a batch of defatted chicken broth and made the ice cubes as suggested in the Rice Day section (see page 28), you can throw a couple of the chicken-broth ice cubes into the wok and stir-fry in this. Oil, olive oil included, has between 120 and 140 calories per tablespoon. You save a lot of calories—up to 10 percent of your daily intake—when you use the defatted chicken broth. (Even though olive oil is healthy, it's best to leave it alone during this maximum weight-loss portion of this diet.

Use small amounts of olive oil in the Lifestyle phase of the 1-Day-at-a-Time diet.)

Another way of cooking your vegetables in the evening is in a large, high-walled cast-iron skillet. You can use some tomato paste or tomato juice as a base for cooking a vegetable stew. This works well using sliced or canned tomatoes, onions, zucchini, and eggplant. This is my version of a ratatouille. It is wonderful and easy to prepare. So is the Ratatouille recipe included here.

Recipes for Vegetable Day

Ratatouille

          3 medium onions, thinly sliced
          2 tablespoons chicken stock, no-salt-added tomato juice, or water
          1 medium eggplant, peeled and cubed
          3 large tomatoes, peeled and cut up
  3 or 4 zucchini, cubed
          3 green peppers, cut in small strips
        ½ lb. mushrooms, sliced
          1 6-oz. can tomato paste
          2 cloves garlic, mashed
          1 teaspoon Italian seasoning
        ½ teaspoon dillweed
        ½ teaspoon oregano
        ¼ teaspoon white pepper
          1 bay leaf
        ¼ teaspoon grated lemon rind
          1 tablespoon Angostura bitters (optional)

In a large nonstick skillet, sauté onions in chicken stock, unsalted tomato juice, or water until translucent. Add remaining ingredients while stirring lightly. Place in baking dish. Cover loosely with foil and bake in 350°F. oven for 40 minutes. (Some of the liquid will evaporate.) Remove bay leaf. Yields 4 servings.

Zucchini-Lettuce Salad

½ head lettuce (iceberg, green leaf, or red leaf), broken into bite-size pieces

½ head romaine, broken into bite-size pieces

2 zucchini, thinly sliced

½ cup thinly sliced radishes

3 green onions, sliced

½ cup wine vinegar, tarragon vinegar, or no-oil salad dressing

Toss all vegetables together. Pour vinegar over the salad and toss. Yields 6 servings.

Cucumbers in Yogurt

3 cucumbers, peeled and sliced

1 cup plain nonfat yogurt

1 teaspoon dillweed

⅛ teaspoon white pepper

Place sliced cucumbers in serving bowl and toss with yogurt, dill, and pepper. Chill and serve. Yields 4 servings.

Stir-Fry Veggies

3 tablespoons chicken broth
3 ribs celery, finely sliced
2 carrots, cut into matchsticks
1 lb. broccoli, cut in flowerets with stems sliced
1 cup sliced mushrooms
   Any other seasonal vegetable desired
1 teaspoon grated lemon rind
1 clove garlic, mashed in garlic press
½ teaspoon ground ginger

In a large nonstick skillet, heat chicken broth over medium heat. Add all remaining ingredients. Stir-fry for 5–6 minutes or until vegetables are tender. Yields 4–6 servings.

Zucchini Italiano

3 tablespoons chicken broth
2 medium onions, sliced into rings
2 cloves garlic, minced
1 teaspoon crushed oregano leaves
¼ teaspoon crushed basil leaves
1 6-oz. can tomato paste
¼ cup water
2 lbs. zucchini, cut into ½-inch slices

In a nonstick skillet, combine chicken broth, onions, garlic, oregano, and basil. Cook until onions are tender. Add tomato paste, water, and zucchini. Cover and cook over low heat for 20 minutes, stirring occasionally. Yields 6–8 servings.

Green Beans and Mushrooms

1½ cups sliced mushrooms
 2 tablespoons water
 2 teaspoons dry sherry
 ⅛ teaspoon ground nutmeg
 ¼ teaspoon ground majoram
 1 10-oz. package frozen cut green beans or ¾ lb. fresh
    green beans
    Cherry tomatoes, cut in halves

Place the mushrooms in a medium-size nonstick skillet with 2 tablespoons water. Cook 2–3 minutes. Stir in sherry, nutmeg, and marjoram. Add green beans and simmer, covered, for 10 minutes. Garnish with cherry tomatoes. Yields 4 servings.

Stuffed Pattypan Squash

6–10 pattypan squash (light-green summer squash)
   1 10-oz. package frozen mixed vegetables

Steam squash until tender. While squash is steaming, cook mixed vegetables according to package directions. Scoop out cooked squash, leaving a shell about ½ inch thick. Combine squash pulp with drained vegetables. Fill squash shell with vegetable mixture. Yields 6 servings.

Stir-Fry Broccoli

1½ lbs. fresh broccoli, cut in flowerets with stems sliced
    thinly
 4 carrots, cut into matchsticks

1 cup sliced mushrooms

¼ cup sliced onion

2 tablespoons water

1 cup fresh bean sprouts

2 teaspoons cornstarch

1 cup chicken broth

1 clove garlic, minced

¼ teaspoon ground ginger

Scant ⅛ teaspoon white pepper

1 red pepper, cut into strips

In a large nonstick skillet, combine broccoli, carrots, mushrooms, onion, and 2 tablespoons water. Stir-fry over medium heat for about 3–4 minutes. Add bean sprouts. Stir cornstarch into a little cold water in a measuring cup. Add enough chicken broth to make 1 cup. Add to vegetable mixture along with garlic, ginger, and white pepper. Simmer about 3 minutes, stirring, until liquid thickens and vegetables are tender-crisp. Garnish with red pepper strips. Yields 4 servings.

Squash Souffle

2 cups cooked millet (cook according to directions on package)

*1 large banana squash, peeled

2 carrots, peeled

½ clove garlic

1 teaspoon fresh lemon juice

½ teaspoon cinnamon

* *Variation:* Substitute broccoli, asparagus, or other green vegetables of your choice.

¼ teaspoon white pepper

4 egg whites

Pam or Mazola nonstick cooking spray

Steam the squash and carrots for 20 minutes. Preheat oven to 325°F.

Place the vegetables in a blender. Add garlic, lemon juice, cinnamon, and pepper. Blend until smooth.

In a separate bowl, beat the egg white until stiff peaks form. Gently fold in the squash mixture.

Spray an 11 × 14 × 2-inch nonstick baking pan with cooking spray. Place the cooked millet in the bottom of the pan. Pour the squash mixture over the millet. Bake in a 325°F. oven for 20–25 minutes. Yields 6 servings as an entree or 8 as a side dish.

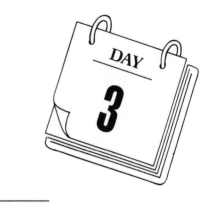

PASTA DAY

Did you know that good pasta is one of the finest diet foods in the world? It may be difficult to believe that a delicious pasta with a zesty tomato sauce, or gourmet pasta with garlic and herbs, is an excellent complex carbohydrate perfectly in keeping with the principles of the 1-Day-at-a-Time diet. There are many flavorful and wholesome varieties of pasta, including whole-wheat and spinach—and besides wonderful tastes that will satisfy a gourmet, pasta will give you sustained energy without weight gain.

It isn't necessary to use lots of oil or butter to make a great pasta meal. Healthy pasta sauce is easy and fast to prepare, as you will see in the recipe section of this book (see page 161) and at the end of this chapter (see page 46). Pasta, prepared without oil, butter, or any meat is one of the least fattening foods you can eat. As a satisfying and appetite-suppressing food, pasta is an important part of any weight-loss and weight-maintenance diet.

The slow and steady absorption of complex carbohydrates (like pasta) into the bloodstream eliminates the low blood sugar that sets up a desire for more fattening foods. This is how Pasta Day can help to satisfy your appetite, and you will still lose weight.

Two Hundred Varieties of Pasta

There are innumerable varieties of pasta to choose from, as well as a tremendous number of healthy ways to prepare pasta with wonderful sauces. Pasta is versatile, easy to cook, and nutritious. Whole-wheat pasta is healthier than the regular white-flour kind. Try the whole-wheat pasta available at health-food stores. If the taste doesn't appeal to you, you can alternate it with the regular pasta that you buy in the grocery store. You can use linguini, spaghetti, angel hair, tortellini, curly-cues, or whatever variety you like.

You should limit the amount of pasta that you eat on Pasta Day to three-quarters of a pound (uncooked). This yields about six cups cooked pasta.

One of my 1-Day-at-a-Time seminar participants said that she couldn't even finish all of the pasta allowed on this day. Did you ever think you'd be on a diet where you'd be allowed more pasta than you can eat?

As a variation on Pasta Day you can substitute spaghetti squash for the pasta (see the Pasta Pretender recipe, page 246).

How to Cook Pasta

For any amount of pasta, boil about three times as much water as the amount of pasta (the more water the better). Slowly add the pasta so that the water does not stop boiling. Cook for about 6 to 10 minutes, or until the pasta is still a bit firm ("al dente"). Drain the pasta, then run cold water over it for a few seconds to eliminate sticking. Drain again, add the Marinara Sauce described below or one in the recipe section, and enjoy!

What to Put on the Pasta

If you want to use a marinara sauce it must be made without oil. You can use your own recipe, or the Marinara Sauce recipe in this book (see pages 46 and 227). The main sauce for Pasta Day must be a tomato-based marinara sauce without oil, but it can have lots of garlic in it if you desire. Or you can make a primavera sauce with lots of chopped vegetables; that's a mix and match that's allowable on Pasta Day.

There are four acceptable pasta sauces that I know of available in health-food stores, each made without oil: Johnston's, Robbie's, Pritikin, and Weight Watchers. You can add mushrooms, either fresh or bottled mushrooms that have been drained, to the spaghetti sauce to give it a tasty, meaty texture.

Mix and Match with Cottage Cheese

Another mix and match idea is to combine some nonfat cottage cheese with the pasta. You can bake it as a noodle kugel (see recipe section for a fabulous recipe). Weight Watchers low-fat cottage cheese is acceptable whenever cottage cheese is mentioned in this book.

Experiment with fresh herbs on your pasta. Try fresh basil, diced or chopped, which adds a wonderful pungent taste to tomato sauces. Basil should be added to tomato sauce at the last minute to impart the strongest taste.

Try other herbs such as parsley, dill, tarragon, oregano, or marjoram on your pasta dishes. You can buy jars of "Italian seasoning" herbs in any market; these herbs are a perfect blend for use in many sauces, combined with garlic and any fresh herbs that may be available.

Pasta for Breakfast?

While some of you may think that having pasta for breakfast is a bit out of the ordinary, most of my patients who have tried it love it. After all, breakfast cereals are made of the same thing that whole-wheat pasta is made from. Those of you who are a little timid about having pasta for breakfast can substitute an egg-white omelette or hard-boiled egg whites (see Protein Day, pages 65 and 66).

Recipe for Pasta Day

Marinara Sauce

    *2 tablespoons extra-virgin olive oil
     3 cups chopped onions
     4 cloves garlic, chopped
     2 cups diced carrots (about 5 or 6)
   **6 cups chopped fresh tomatoes (or canned, drained well)
     4 tablespoons dried basil, or 3 tablespoons fresh basil
        White pepper to taste
        Water

Heat oil in a large saucepan or skillet; add onions, garlic, and carrots. Sauté until onions begin to brown. Add tomatoes, basil, and white pepper. Cover and simmer 15 minutes. Pour sauce into food processor or blender 2 cups at a time and puree to a creamy consistency. Return to pan and stir in water ¼ cup at a time until desired consistency. Cover and simmer for 10 minutes. Yields 6 servings.

  * Omit olive oil during Jump-Start phase and sauté in nonstick pan using Pam or Mazola cooking spray.
 ** About 12 large Roma tomatoes, or use tomatoes of your choice.

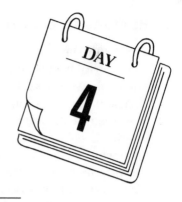

FRUIT DAY

The United States is blessed by being a very commercial nation—it engages in trade with countries all over the world. So we can walk into the supermarket in the middle of January, when there is snow on the ground, and see fresh peaches, strawberries, watermelon, and all kinds of exotic fruits. Even bananas, mangoes, and papayas that come from tropical or semitropical climates can be purchased while we are in the middle of a winter snowstorm. Fruits are generally warm-country products, and one of the advantages of eating fruit in a warm climate is that it helps to dissipate heat from the body. In other words, fruits are cooling, so if you start the 1-Day-at-a-Time diet in the middle of a cold winter, it might be best not to include the Fruit or the Juice Day in your Jump-Start cycles. Fruit Day and Juice Day are best accomplished when the weather is warmer.

What Fruits to Eat on Fruit Day

On Fruit Day you can eat up to 12 fruits. Watermelon is a wonderful fruit to include. Watermelon not only has a great natural sweetness, but is also full of water and low in calories. It acts as a diuretic and helps stimulate the kidneys because of its water content. Watermelon makes a wonderful breakfast fruit. You can pretty much eat as much watermelon as you want for breakfast and that only counts as one fruit. Any other melon will make a great breakfast fruit too. Half of a honeydew melon, or half a cantaloupe, counts as one fruit. Other melons, such as casaba and crenshaw, are also quite acceptable.

You don't have to eat melon for breakfast; you could eat an orange, an apple, a banana, or one of each of those if you wish. Or you could make a fruit salad using melons, strawberries, banana, pineapple, apple, or other fruits. A cup of berries or half a cup of grapes counts as one fruit.

On Fruit Day you can essentially eat fruit all day long to keep your hunger satisfied. It is best to eat one or two pieces of fruit at a time and not overindulge and stuff yourself with fruit. (If you eat large amounts of fruit at one time you may develop intestinal gas.) The important thing about Fruit Day is that you eat *nothing but fresh fruit*; it is relatively low in calories and high in water content and fiber content. Peaches, pears, apricots, and nectarines are all acceptable fruits for Fruit Day. *Dried fruit is not allowed.* Dried fruit is too dense in concentrated calories because all the water is removed; too much sugar remains, which will stimulate insulin production and cause you to get hungry and thus gain weight.

Precaution for diabetics: because fruit has so much sugar (this caution also goes for Juice Day) it may contribute to raising your blood sugar and changing your medication requirement on Fruit Day. If you have diabetes, it is recommended that you not include Fruit Day or Juice Day as part of the 1-Day-at-a-Time diet.

Mix and Match on Fruit Day

One of the mix and matches you can do on Fruit Day is to put a scoop of *nonfat* vanilla frozen yogurt in half a cantaloupe for an evening snack. Another mix and match for Fruit Day is to put a little nonfat cottage cheese in half a cantaloupe. You can choose honeydew, crenshaw, or casaba instead—or one of the yuppie melons that cost a bundle—but use only nonfat yogurt or low-fat or nonfat cottage cheese.

Recipes for Fruit Day

Fruit Medley*

1 apple, cut into bite-size pieces

2 oranges, peeled and sliced

2 bananas, peeled and sliced

2 ripe pears (Bosc, Comice, or Anjou), cut into bite-size pieces

1 cup black or purple grapes, seeded and halved

½ cup fresh-squeezed orange juice (remove seeds, do not strain)

Combine fruit and toss lightly. Combine orange juice and wine. Pour over fruit and mix gently to coat the fruit. Chill at least 2 hours. Yields 6–8 servings.

* Counts as ten fruits on fruit day.

Fruit Compote

1 large banana, sliced
1 cup plain nonfat yogurt
1 cup fresh pineapple, diced
1 cup diced melon of your choice
6 large strawberries with stems left on

Place banana and yogurt in a blender and blend until smooth. Put equal amounts of pineapple and melon in dessert cups and spoon the banana-yogurt mixture over the fruit. Garnish each serving with a strawberry. Yields 6 generous servings.

No-Cooking Applesauce

1 tablespoon fresh lemon juice
⅛ teaspoon cardamom
⅛ teaspoon ground cinnamon
4 medium-large apples, peeled, cored, and quartered

In blender or food processor, place lemon juice, cardamom, cinnamon, and half of the apples. Blend until mixture looks like applesauce. Gradually add the remaining apples and blend until smooth. Yields 2½–3 cups.

Melon Garni

1 cantaloupe
1 tablespoon lemon juice
1 cup seedless grapes
1 cup watermelon balls

Other fruit, such as strawberries, cherries, or other types of melon may be substituted

Cut cantaloupe in half, preserving a one-inch-wide strip connected at each side to serve as the handle of a basket-shaped shell formed by the rind. Scoop out the flesh of the cantaloupe, maintaining the basket shape. Coat the inside of the cantaloupe with lemon juice, saving any extra. Combine fruit in the shell. Pour any remaining lemon juice over the mixture. Chill until ready to serve. Yields 6 servings.

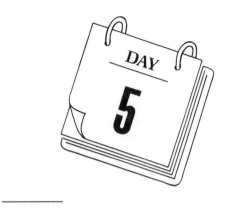

POTATO DAY

The potato is a source of concentrated complex carbohydrate and is full of energy. In addition potatoes are filling, and you will be able to lose weight easily eating nothing but potatoes on Potato Day, and you will not be hungry. Potatoes are fun! However, just as salad dressing sometimes has more calories than the salad itself, you must also be careful of what you put on the potato, because the toppings may have more calories than the potato itself.

One of the things you have to be careful of when you shop for potatoes in the supermarket is to avoid potatoes that are sprouted. The sprouting potato has an increased content of solanine, a toxic substance that in large quantities can even be fatal. Some potatoes are high in solanine even when they have only a small amount of sprouts. If you notice a green hue just under the skin, the potato is rich in solanine and should not be eaten. Apparently the potato produces solanine in response to stress.

On Potato Day you may eat a total of up to eight potatoes: one or two at each meal; one between each meal; and, if you have any left, one between dinner and bedtime. You don't have to eat that many, but that is the maximum number allowed. Remember, it takes only an hour or so to bake a potato in a conventional oven, and less time than that to boil potatoes. A microwave is even faster.

How to Bake a Potato

I'm sure many of you cooks know how to prepare potatoes just as well as I do, but let me run through the way that I usually prepare them. A lot depends on how your oven bakes, but the best temperature for baking potatoes is somewhere between 400 and 500°F., and the duration of time is somewhere between 50 minutes and 75 minutes, depending on the size of the potato. Each of you will have to determine the exact time with your own oven. You can bake white and red potatoes, but we are talking about russet baking potatoes here.

If you prepare the potatos the night before so that they'll be ready for breakfast, I suggest that you cook them only for about 45 minutes. You might want to partially bake two to four potatoes the night before you start Potato Day. What do you do with the partially baked potatoes? There are lots of options.

Potatoes for Breakfast

One option is to simply finish baking the potato in the morning. You can complete the last 15 minutes of baking in a conventional oven, or you can put the potato in the microwave and zap it on high temperature for about 6 to 8 minutes. Another option is to slice the partially baked potato into four or eight slices and toast them in a toaster oven until browned on top. Then eat the potato slices as finger food. Another option is to slice your partially cooked potato thinly and fry it in a Teflon nonstick fry pan at a relatively low heat to give the potato a chance to finish cooking and to brown on each side. Again, you end up with a potato that is crispy and can be eaten as finger food, or you can eat it from a plate for lunch or dinner and add a small amount of ketchup or mustard.

Yet another option is to do like the Irish do and instead of using russet potatoes, use small new potatoes. Boil them in water for 12 to 15 minutes, then mash the potatoes in a little bit of skim milk. Or simply cut them up and eat a plate for breakfast. See "What to Put on the Potatoes," below.

For those of you who feel you need protein in the morning, a trusty egg-white omelette is acceptable for breakfast on Potato Day. Take some partially cooked potatoes, dice them and throw them into your nonstick fry pan, brown them, and pour in the egg whites to make an egg-white potato frittata.

What to Put on the Potatoes

One of the toppings you can put on your baked potato is a product called Molly McButter. Molly McButter is carried in the spice and condiment section of the supermarket and has four calories per serving. It has 90 milligrams of salt per serving, but that shouldn't be a problem for many of you. There are three flavors: sour cream, cheese, and plain butter. You can use as much Molly McButter on your potato as a seasoning as you like, and it does give it a taste of real butter at a minimum number of calories. You may like the sour cream flavor just as well; it too has only four calories per serving and is delicious. My favorite is the cheese flavored.

Several other products are similar to Molly McButter. McCormick makes an imitation butter sprinkle, Best o' Butter, which also has four calories per serving and is quite tasty. McCormick also has a cheese-flavored sprinkle that has six calories per serving, and it too is a low-calorie alternative for potato seasoning. Butter Buds and Instead of Butter are also acceptable sprinkles.

The recipe for Mock Sour Kream (see pages 56 and 225) is another totally acceptable topping. You can add a few chopped chives and enjoy a delicious, healthy, extremely low-fat topping for your baked potato.

Another acceptable topping is salsa or picante sauce.

Potatoes for Lunch

For lunch you also have a multitude of options. Many shopping malls have fast-food stands that sell baked potatoes, and you can get a plain baked potato. I take a little bottle of Molly McButter when I go out for a baked potato.

If you don't have someone to bake your potatoes for you, then you have to take your own partially baked potatoes and find a microwave. You may have one in your office. Most 7-Eleven stores and other convenience stores have a microwave. My experience has been that they don't mind if you come in and use their microwave for a few minutes. You could bring in your partially cooked baked potato and finish cooking it in the microwave.

Snacking and Dinner on Potato Day

If you get hungry between your potato meals, you can have a few carrot sticks, celery sticks, or other raw vegetables as always. For dinner you can use some of the options we mentioned for breakfast: baked potato, boiled potato, roasted potato, or egg-white potato frittata. You can also have potato soup (see page 61 in the chapter on Soup Day), equal to two potatoes if you use it on Potato Day.

Another splendid way of preparing potatoes is to slice them and cook them in the toaster oven as mentioned above. You can do this with a partially cooked baked potato or with a totally raw potato. When you use a raw potato you have to slice it much thinner. You can put the potato slices on a piece of aluminum foil that has been sprayed with one of the nonstick cooking sprays, such as Pam or Mazola, to prevent the potatoes from sticking to the foil. You have to watch them; again, cooking time depends on the idiosyncrasies of your toaster oven. When they get brown and crispy on the top, turn them over and brown and crisp them on the other side. If you have cut them thin enough, they will be done in the middle and taste like delicious French fries. Between dinner and bedtime, a left-over cold baked potato makes a wonderful snack, and it keeps you kosher on Potato Day.

Potato Skins

What about the potato skins? If there is no green solanine visible underneath, then the potato skins may be eaten if they have been well scrubbed; however, sometimes there is just a little bit of solanine that can't be seen. My experience is that if you eat too many potato skins on Potato Day, it may upset your stomach. You will have to see what your response is. I suggest that you don't eat more than two or three potato skins a day. The skins on new potatoes, which are better for boiling, don't seem to have as much solanine and are quite acceptable. White and red potatoes make solanine too, so you have to watch out for any green color showing through. Don't use green or sprouted white or red potatoes.

Recipes for Potato Day

Mock Sour Kream

   1 cup dry-curd or low-fat cottage cheese
   ¼ cup nonfat skim milk
   ½ teaspoon fresh lemon juice

Combine ingredients in a blender and blend until smooth. If consistency is too thick, add more milk a teaspoon at a time until desired thickness is achieved. Use for dips. Mix your own blend of herbs and spices. Season with chives or onions and serve over baked potatoes. Yields approximately 1½ cups.

Homemade Picante Sauce

  3 large tomatoes, cubed
  1 6-oz. can tomato puree
  ¼ teaspoon minced garlic
  3 tablespoons fresh cilantro
  3 whole green chiles (not jalapeños)

Combine ingredients in food processor and process until chunky. Store in refrigerator. Yields 1 cup.

Stuffed Baked Potatoes

  4 medium baking potatoes
  1 cup dry-curd or nonfat cottage cheese
  ¼ cup plain nonfat yogurt
  1 tablespoon nonfat milk (or more for desired consistency)
  ½ cup finely chopped onion
  2 tablespoons water
  ⅛ teaspoon white pepper
    Chopped chives

Bake well-scrubbed potatoes in a 450°F. oven for 1 hour. Mash the cottage cheese with yogurt and milk. Mix well. Sauté onion in 2 tablespoons water in a nonstick skillet until tender. Cut a thin slice off the top of each potato. Remove the pulp and save the shell. Combine cottage cheese mixture with pepper, onion, and potato pulp. Mash. Stuff the potato mixture into the shells. Reheat the potatoes in a 350°F. oven until hot. Sprinkle with chopped chives before serving. Yields 4 servings.

Oven French Fries

2 large potatoes
2 egg whites, beaten
   Dillweed, crushed

Preheat oven to 425°F. Peel and cut potatoes into wedges. Dip the wedges into beaten egg whites and sprinkle with dill. Bake on a nonstick pan at 425°F. for 25–30 minutes. Yields 2 servings.

Karen's Crusty Broiler-Fried Potatoes

Bake 1 potato in microwave for 10 minutes (or in conventional oven for 1 hour at 450°F. Cool and slice as thinly as possible. Line broiler with foil. Crush one garlic clove and brush garlic across foil (optional). Spray foil lightly with Pam or Mazola nonstick cooking spray. Broil potato slices on high for 5–7 minutes a side. Delicious! Yields 1 serving.

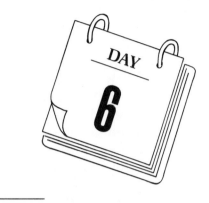

SOUP DAY

Of all the Jump-Start days of the 1-Day-at-a-Time diet, my personal favorite is Soup Day. Eating soup is one of the easiest ways to lose weight. Soup is tasty, there are many varieties available, and it's extremely nutritious, filling, and relatively easy to prepare.

I recommend that you make your own soup using my mother's recipe at the end of this chapter (see page 62). If you decide to use store-bought soup, my recommendation is that you buy it in a health-food store or health-food section of any good market. The Health Valley line is particularly tasty and made with only healthy ingredients. It is available in a salt-free variety, and I strongly urge you to try that. The two ingredients that you have to be careful of in commercial soups are fat and salt. An average can of soup from the supermarket has at least a gram of sodium, and on the 1-Day-at-a-Time diet eating soup with that much sodium is prohibited. Sometimes commercial canners do restrict the salt content, but in reading the labels of many of these salt-restricted commercial soups, I find that there is often a great deal of fat in the soup. This gives the soup a creamy, luscious flavor, but this fat is also prohibited on the 1-Day-at-a-Time diet.

Health Valley, however, has been able to combine herbs and natural spices in a way that makes their soups very tasty and salt free. The oil that they use is a healthy oil and it's not used in excess. If you don't like the taste of salt-free soups, you can add small amounts of salt or soy sauce. Because they have done such a good job with the herbs and spices, it takes very little salt to make the soup tasty. My favorite variety of the Health Valley line is the potato-leek soup, which you can also try on Potato Day as well as Soup Day. It is absolutely delicious. I'll often take a can of the Health Valley salt-free potato soup, put it in a styrofoam cup at the office and heat it in the microwave for five minutes and have a hot cup of soup for lunch. It's satisfying, nourishing, tasty, and a whole can has only 220 calories.

Other brands of soup in the health-food store that are low in fat and sodium include Pritikin and Hain. Hain makes both a salted and a salt-free variety; you should use the salt-free. Pritikin makes only low-sodium soups.

Edythe's Fresh Vegetable Soup

The best approach, however, is to make your own. If you use as many vegetables as possible you will create a truly nutritious low-calorie soup. Edythe's Fresh Vegetable Soup recipe on pages 62 and 196 is delicious and easy to make.

When you make this vegetable soup you should prepare at least 10 quarts at a time. You can freeze it in quart-size, air-tight containers and always have it available at a moment's notice.

To help flavor your soup stock you can use some of those chicken-broth ice cubes that we mentioned earlier for seasoning rice and for seasoning stir-fry vegetables in your wok (see page 28).

How Much Soup Can You Eat?

The amount of soup you can eat on Soup Day will depend in part on whether it is store-bought or homemade. If it is homemade garden vegetable soup from the recipe below, you can eat all you want. Remember, you have to prepare ahead of time for Soup Day because the soup has to be ready for breakfast. Although you may not have thought of having soup for breakfast before, it is a wonderful, hearty, nourishing way to start the day, especially in the wintertime. For those of you too timid to try soup for breakfast, the egg-white omelette/vegetable frittata is an acceptable alternative.

You really can eat all you want of this homemade vegetable soup. It will be filling, and you will still lose weight. If you use store-bought canned soups such as the Health Valley brand, you must limit yourself to four cans a day —one can for breakfast, one for lunch, one for dinner, and one can as a snack. You can also have your raw vegetables in between as a snack without concern.

In addition to potato-leek soup, Health Valley has a mushroom-barley soup that is quite delicious. The "no added salt" lentil soup, black bean soup, and five-bean soup are each delicious, but they have a few more calories than the potato or mushroom-barley. You must still limit yourself to four cans of soup per day if you use the beans or lentil soups. These do provide excellent fiber and have more protein than the other soups. If you feel the need for additional protein when you make your homemade soup, you can always add one skin-free, fat-free chicken breast to the 10 quarts of vegetable soup. As the chicken meat cooks down, its flavor will permeate the soup and it will provide that little extra protein that some of you might need.

On Soup Day you can eat just one soup like the vegetable soup all day long, or you can mix and match different kinds of soup.

If you make your own bean, lentil, or pea soup you have

to limit the amount you eat in a day because of its higher caloric content compared to the vegetable soup. Restrict your intake to a maximum of four servings of 12 ounces each.

Recipes for Soup Day

Edythe's Fresh Vegetable Soup

4 cups Seasoned Chicken Broth (see page 189) or water
3 cloves garlic, minced
1 medium zucchini, sliced
1 turnip, diced
1 10-oz. package frozen corn kernels
2 large onions, chopped
1 cup diced carrots
1 cup cut-up broccoli
1 small eggplant, peeled and cubed
1 16-oz. can unsalted tomatoes, mashed
½ teaspoon ground coriander
⅛ teaspoon white pepper
1 bay leaf
1 teaspoon basil

In a soup pot, bring chicken broth or water to a boil. Reduce heat. Add remaining ingredients. Bring back to a boil. Reduce to simmer and simmer, with lid slightly ajar, 10 minutes or until vegetables are barely tender. Remove bay leaf. Yields 6 servings.

Gazpacho

    1 quart no-salt-added tomato juice or no-salt-added V8
      juice, chilled
    2 tablespoons wine vinegar
    1 clove garlic
    ½ green pepper, cut in pieces
    1 medium zucchini
    1 rib celery, cut in pieces
    2 ripe tomatoes
    ½ small onion
    ½ teaspoon dried basil
    ¼ teaspoon white pepper
    3 teaspoons chopped parsley

Use the chopping blade in the bowl of your food processor. Start with 2 cups of tomato juice. Add remaining ingredients and process until well blended. Add
1 more cup of tomato juice and process until well
blended. Pour the remaining tomato juice and the
blended mixture into a 1½-quart container. Stir. Chill
for several hours. If you are in a hurry to serve, pour
into serving dishes with an ice cube in each dish.
Garnish with chopped parsley. Yields 6 (8-oz.) servings.

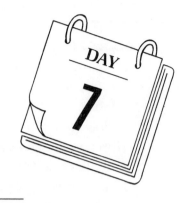

PROTEIN DAY

Most Americans eat too much protein. It is extremely important to balance the amount of protein in your diet on a day-to-day basis for optimum health. The "Eat Moderate Amounts of Protein" chapter in the Lifestyle phase section of this book (see page 124) provides the rationale and details for healthy protein nutrition.

The protein requirement varies from person to person; some people feel that they need extra protein in order to maintain their strength. The purpose of Protein Day on the 1-Day-at-a-Time diet is to give you insight as to how to eat protein in a healthy manner. This day gives you an opportunity to learn ways of incorporating healthy protein into your diet without getting excess amounts of cholesterol and unhealthy fats.

Breakfast on Protein Day

On Protein Day you'll start with an egg-white omelette or hard-boiled egg whites for breakfast. The whites have all of the egg's protein and none of the cholesterol or fat.

On a recent trip to Las Vegas I was delighted to see an egg-white omelette on the menu at the Golden Nugget. When I called room service to order it, I inquired as to how they prepare it. They informed me that they knew exactly how to prepare it, because Mr. Rickles (Don Rickles) orders the egg-white omelette all the time.

How to Cook an Egg-White Omelette

To prepare your egg whites you simply separate the whites from the yolks; this can be done by decanting the egg back and forth between the shells, and then simply discard the yolk. In the "Understanding Fats and Cholesterol" section of the Lifestyle phase of the 1-Day-at-a-Time diet we discuss the egg/cholesterol issue in more detail (see page 109).

It is best to use a Teflon nonstick frying pan for the omelette. You have to take care of the pan properly by using plastic or wooden utensils only. You don't want to scratch the Teflon so that particles come off and get into your food.

Often I have a wonderful egg-white omelette made with two mushrooms finely chopped, two scallions also chopped, and a small piece of zucchini chopped; all these vegetables are sautéed and browned in a Teflon pan that has been sprayed with a nonstick cooking spray, such as Pam (I prefer the olive oil Pam). Then the egg whites are added. I am also fond of this egg-white omelette with sliced water chestnuts, which you can buy in a can. When the water chestnuts are drained and sautéed they crisp up and add a crunchy consistency to the omelette that is truly delicious. If you don't have fresh mushrooms you can use canned as long as you drain them well. If you don't drain them completely, the liquid they add to the fry pan will cause the hot olive oil to splatter, and that's dangerous. You don't have to use scallions; you can use red, white, or regular onions chopped and sautéed. Green pepper, yellow squash, and tomatoes can also be sautéed for your omelette. Use as many egg whites as you like; three or four is not too much for this meal. If you use a lot of vegetables, you may find that two egg whites are enough to fill up the pan.

One of my patients loved the egg-white omelette so much that she made it daily; she created her own Mix and Match Day using large quantities of vegetables and 10 to 12 egg whites per day, making three or four meals of omelettes, varying the vegetables each time. She would eat other raw vegetables between meals as a snack. *Her weight loss averaged more than a pound a day over these days.* She felt terrific, satisfied, and was never hungry. The egg-white omelette with lots of vegetables is a dish that you can always come back to as a healthy, delicious, low-calorie, high-protein meal that will invariably satiate your appetite.

Hard-Boiled Egg Whites

Another easy way to prepare your egg whites is by boiling them. Two to four (or more) hard-boiled egg whites will make a filling, nutritious, high-protein breakfast on Protein Day.

How to prepare hard-boiled egg whites: Place the eggs in a saucepan and cover them with cold tap water. Place the pan on the stove over medium heat for 20 minutes. The water won't start boiling right away, but that's okay. Bringing the temperature of the eggs up slowly may prevent the shells from cracking during cooking. I often add a pinch of salt to the water; this also helps to keep the shells from cracking. At the end of 20 minutes, remove the pan from the heat. Cool the eggs under tap water before removing the shells. Discard the yolks; eat only the whites.

You can also use egg whites prepared this way as a condiment on your raw vegetable salad for lunch. Egg whites are one of the best cholesterol-free, nonfat protein sources.

Snacking on Protein Day

Although eating nothing but protein all day long is pretty much what the Eskimos do on their fish diet, most Americans would not be happy eating protein all day long. Protein Day is really a Mix and Match day. You won't be snacking on protein—that would be too much protein (see "Eat Moderate Amounts of Protein" on page 124). So the rule on Protein Day is that if you want to have a snack, you can eat raw vegetables all day long.

Lunch on Protein Day

Lunch on Protein Day is a mix and match between vegetables and protein. You are going to have a large salad with lettuce, tomatoes, and other raw vegetables, and you are going to garnish this salad with protein. You have several choices for your protein garnish. One choice would be a small (3.5-oz.) can of water-packed tuna; after draining the water to get rid of most of the salt, you can sprinkle the tuna over the salad. Remember, you can use any of the no-oil reduced-calorie salad dressings (see page 185). Other options to top off your salad on Protein Day are diced chunks of breast of chicken or turkey that has been skinned and defatted; the whites from several hard-boiled eggs; and a 3¾-oz. can of water-packed salmon that has been drained like the tuna. Another option would be to have another egg-white omelette for lunch as you did for breakfast.

You can have all the raw vegetables you want throughout the afternoon.

How Much Protein on Protein Day?

Your total protein intake for the day, excluding the egg whites, will be eight ounces. This could consist of fish or defatted and skinned breast of turkey or chicken. You can split this up however you like between lunch and dinner. If you have two to three ounces for lunch, then you can have five or six ounces for dinner—or vice versa if you prefer to eat more protein at lunch than at dinner. Tuna and salmon must be packed in water instead of oil. If you use canned sardines you must drain off all of the oil. Do not use boneless and skinless sardines, because the bones (as well as the bones in salmon) are an excellent source of calcium. Fresh fish is always acceptable.

Dinner on Protein Day

For dinner you have the same options you had at lunch plus a few more. Like the lady who enjoyed the egg-white omelettes with vegetables so much, you could have another omelette for dinner. You could broil a piece of fish or a defatted, skinned chicken breast. You can have all the raw vegetable salad you want with no-oil reduced-calorie salad dressing to accompany your fish or fowl. The more salad you eat, the more weight you will lose. (See "Eat More Vegetables," page 116). Again, if you are hungry between dinner and bedtime, your snack on Protein Day is raw vegetables.

Avoid Beans and Peas on Protein Day

Legumes such as beans and peas are extremely good sources of vegetable protein. However, they are not recommended in Jump-Start because of their high calorie count. Animal protein from fish and chicken is a much more efficient source of protein. This means that you get lots more protein for fewer calories. For that reason I don't recommend the incorporation of beans, peas, and other legumes as sources of protein during Protein Day. During the Lifestyle phase of this diet, small amounts of beans and peas can be eaten, especially when combined with whole grains to give a terrific source of protein that is totally cholesterol free and extremely low in fat.

Recipes for Protein Day

Basic Broiled Fish

Rinse fish quickly in cold water and pat dry with a paper towel. Squeeze a generous amount of lemon juice on fish 20–30 minutes before broiling. Preheat broiling pan for at least 10 minutes to broiling heat (approx. 550°F.). Place fish on preheated broiling rack. Broil fillets and steaks 2 inches from flame; broil split fish and whole dressed fish 2–6 inches from flame. Broil about 20 minutes per inch of thickness at the thickest part of the fish. (A good average thickness for fillets is 1 inch.)

Baked Flounder

Place rinsed fish in a glass baking dish. Mix ⅓ cup white wine, 1 tablespoon chopped parsley, and 2 teaspoons lemon juice. Pour mixture over the fish. Bake uncovered at 425°F. for 12–15 minutes or until fish flakes with a fork.

Broiled Sole Fillets

For extra good flavor, squeeze lemon juice on fish about 15–20 minutes before broiling. Baste fillets with mashed garlic and lemon juice. Broil for 10–12 minutes or until fish flakes with a fork. Broil thin fillets very near the flame to brown quickly.

Baked Halibut

Place halibut in a glass baking dish. Combine ¼ cup dry white wine with 1 tablespoon lemon juice and pour over the fish. Bake uncovered at 350°F. for 25–30 minutes or until fish flakes with a fork. Sprinkle with chopped parsley about 4–5 minutes before serving.

Salmon is also good baked this way. If possible, use the tail end of the salmon—it is meatier and has fewer small bones.

Chicken and Orange Sauce

    6 chicken breasts, skinned, all visible fat removed
    1 cup sliced mushrooms
    ½ cup fresh-squeezed orange juice
    1 teaspoon grated orange rind
    ½ cup chicken stock
    1 scant teaspoon ground ginger
    1 tablespoon low-salt soy sauce
    ½ cup water
    2 tablespoons cornstarch
    3 tablespoons finely chopped parsley

Arrange chicken breasts in a glass baking dish. Place sliced mushrooms over chicken. Combine orange juice, orange rind, chicken stock, ginger, soy sauce, and water. Pour over chicken and mushrooms. Bake at 350°F. for 45 minutes. Remove from oven, baste the chicken and mushrooms with liquid from baking dish. Remove the chicken and mushrooms from the baking dish; keep them warm. In a saucepan, combine cornstarch with the remaining juices. Heat and stir until sauce is thickened. Pour over chicken and mushrooms. Garnish with chopped parsley. If desired, serve over cooked vegetables. Yields 6 servings.

Chicken Breasts and Mushroom Sauce

4–5 chicken breasts, halved, boned, skinned, all visible fat removed

1 cup chicken broth

¼ cup Sauterne wine

1 tablespoon tomato paste

1 clove garlic, minced

2 tablespoons minced onion

1 tablespoon soy sauce

1 teaspoon dry mustard

2 tablespoons cornstarch

2 tablespoons water

½ lb. fresh mushrooms, sliced

Place chicken breasts in a nonstick skillet. Combine all chicken broth, wine, tomato paste, garlic, onion, soy sauce, and mustard, and pour over the chicken. Cover and cook over low heat for 30 minutes. Dissolve cornstarch in 2 tablespoons water. Stir into skillet. Add mushrooms and continue cooking over low heat for 30 minutes. Yields 4–5 servings.

Boneless Breast of Chicken with Orange and Parsley Sauce

1½ lbs. chicken breasts, boned, skinned, all visible fat removed
 1 bunch green onions with stems, chopped
 1 medium green pepper, chopped
 ½ cup Zante currants (small white raisins)
 ¼ cup lemon juice
 ½ teaspoon ground ginger
 ½ teaspoon ground cloves
 ¼ teaspoon allspice
 1 tablespoon soy sauce
 ½ lb. mushrooms, sliced
 4 tablespoons cornstarch
 ½ cup water
 2 medium oranges, sectioned
 1 cup seedless grapes
 ½ cup chopped parsley

Brown chicken breasts under broiler. In a nonstick skillet, combine onions, green pepper, currants, lemon juice, spices, soy sauce, and chicken. Cover and cook over medium heat for a few minutes. Add mushrooms. Mix cornstarch with ½ cup water and stir into chicken mixture. Stir until thick. Add oranges, grapes, and parsley. Heat for a few minutes and serve over vegetables. Yields 6 servings.

Broiled Chicken Breasts

½ cup dry white wine or water

¼ cup soy sauce, diluted with ¼ cup water

3 cloves garlic, finely minced

2 fingers fresh gingerroot, finely minced

8 chicken breasts, skinned, all visible fat removed

Combine wine or water, diluted soy sauce, garlic, and ginger. Marinate chicken breasts in mixture for at least 2 hours, covered in the refrigerator. Marinate longer if possible. Broil chicken 6 inches from heat, basting often with the marinade, for 20 minutes. Turn and continue broiling and basting 20 minutes longer. May be served hot or cold. Yields 8 servings.

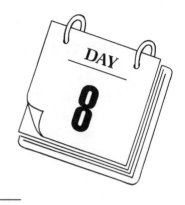

FROZEN YOGURT DAY

Yogurt is one of the healthiest foods I know of. In fact, yogurt is a food that is incorporated into many cultures (pardon the pun) that are known for great longevity. Yogurt is not only high in protein but also one of the best sources of dietary calcium.

Yogurt is made by adding the acidophilus bacteria to milk. The enzymatic action of the bacteria converts the milk into yogurt. When the yogurt is made from nonfat milk—milk that has had the unhealthy butterfat removed—what's left is an excellent source of protein, healthy carbohydrates, and calcium. There seems to be evidence that people who eat yogurt every day live longer, although this is not yet well-substantiated scientific fact.

Frozen Yogurt Day is a fun day on the 1-Day-at-a-Time diet and will provide the insight that you need to choose healthy, low-calorie desserts in the Lifestyle phase.

Over the past few years frozen yogurt stands have sprung up all over the country. In some neighborhoods in Southern

California, there are as many as two or three frozen yogurt stands in a block. The flavors, textures, and quality vary from one yogurt stand to the next, and you will have to find the one that appeals to you best.

The important thing to remember is that you only want *nonfat* frozen yogurt! The difference in calorie count of nonfat frozen yogurt and regular frozen yogurt is significant. Regular frozen yogurt also has fat and cholesterol, which we want to avoid.

Where to Buy Frozen Yogurt

Several yogurt chains have outlets nationwide, and most of them offer nonfat frozen yogurt in a wide range of delicious flavors. You'll have to experiment with the yogurt stands in your area to find your favorites. My personal favorite chains for nonfat frozen yogurt are I Can't Believe It's Yogurt, Heidi's, and Penguins.

Nonfat frozen yogurt will vary in calorie count from about 15 calories per ounce to more than 20 calories per ounce. The extra calories are due to extra nonfat milk and sugar. The amount of nonfat frozen yogurt that you can eat on Yogurt Day will depend on the calorie count of the type you choose.

How Much Frozen Yogurt Can You Eat?

On Frozen Yogurt Day you can have up to 60 ounces (nearly 2 quarts) of nonfat frozen yogurt that has 15 calories per ounce (Heidi's). This will provide 900 calories. If the frozen yogurt has 20 calories per ounce, you must limit yourself to 1½ quarts of frozen yogurt per day. This should be divided over 4 to 6 equal servings.

You have to be careful how you eat your frozen yogurt. Never, never, never eat it straight out of the carton, or you run the risk of making a mistake I have made many times:

eating the whole carton in one sitting. And there it is four o'clock in the afternoon and you have nothing left to eat for the rest of the day. Believe me, that's no fun. So always spoon the yogurt out of the carton into a serving bowl.

Another exciting option on Frozen Yogurt Day is to get the small cake cones that have only about 20 calories each. It's hard to get more than five ounces of yogurt in the cone and piled on top of the cone, so this is an automatic way of limiting your frozen yogurt meal. The 20 calories is a small price to pay to help you limit your yogurt intake at each sitting.

So if you are using 15-calories-per-ounce nonfat frozen yogurt, you can have eight of those cake cones piled with five ounces of yogurt through the course of the day. Many of you may not want to eat that much frozen yogurt. If you use the higher-calorie nonfat yogurt you must reduce the number of servings proportionately.

You don't have to stick to frozen yogurt on Frozen Yogurt Day. You can have plain nonfat yogurt like you buy in the dairy section of the grocery store. Be sure to buy *nonfat* yogurt without added fruit. A quart (32 ounces) is your limit if you choose this option. That is four 8-ounce cartons. Continental Dairy makes a very good nonfat yogurt. Another option is to make your own from our recipe below.

Mix and Match on Frozen Yogurt Day

Most of my weight-loss seminar participants have enjoyed eating frozen yogurt all day long. If, however, you would like to substitute fresh fruit for some of the yogurt and make a Mix and Match Day of it, that's okay too. Be sure to subtract a cup of yogurt from your total yogurt allowance for each fruit.

If you prefer not to have frozen yogurt for breakfast, I suggest that you have an egg-white omelette, hard-boiled egg whites, or fruit.

Under no circumstances should you use the toppings offered in yogurt stores! These are high in calories and unnecessary!

Recipe for Frozen Yogurt Day

Yogurt

1 quart nonfat skim milk

2 acidophilus capsules (available in the health-food section of your supermarket, or in health-food stores), **or**

1 cup plain low-fat yogurt

Scald the milk (do not boil). Add powder from the capsules, or add yogurt.* Let sit in a warm spot in your kitchen overnight. Store in the refrigerator. To make your next batch of yogurt, add a cup of this yogurt to a quart of scalded skim milk. Use the same procedure each time.

* The yogurt as well as the capsules are a source of live acidophilus bacteria, which will convert the milk to yogurt.

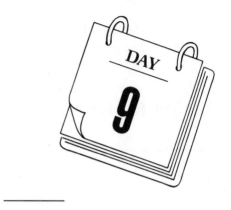

CORN DAY

The Jump-Start phase of this diet is definitely a trick to help you lose weight as painlessly and as quickly as possible. While some people would be totally appalled at a day of eating only corn, others will find it quite tasty, satisfying, appealing, and nutritious too. Corn has been an American staple for hundreds of years. It wouldn't have achieved this status if it were not such a fine, nutritious food. Corn is a high-complex-carbohydrate, relatively low-fat food, and the quality of the fat in it is quite good. If your diet consisted of only corn for long periods of time, you would develop a niacin deficiency. Since you will be taking a B-vitamin supplement with the 1-Day-at-a-Time diet (see page 142), that will not be a problem. The body has sufficient stores of all nutrients to be able to go for a day without any one nutrient, except oxygen.

Ways to Eat Corn

The best way to eat your corn on Corn Day is corn on the cob. It can be prepared relatively quickly by steaming or boiling (see recipe on pages 81 and 239), and it is delicious. Corn is tasty with nothing on it. The succulent, juicy texture is wonderful, and its natural oils give corn a luscious flavor.

Some of the condiments mentioned for Potato Day (see pages 54–55) are acceptable for seasoning your corn, if you choose.

If you buy frozen corn it will take longer to cook; follow the directions on the package. Frozen corn on the cob cooks very nicely in the microwave. On Corn Day you can have up to 12 ears of corn.

In my opinion it is best not to eat canned corn. Stick with the whole ears; otherwise you might get carried away and eat too much. (This is the same principle as taking the frozen yogurt out of the carton on Yogurt Day.) Even though corn is a summer crop, you can get frozen ears of corn in the grocery store all year long. I believe that fresh-frozen corn is better than canned. You can cut the corn off the cob if you want to work with the separate kernels rather than the whole ear. It is best to use a serrated (bread knife) blade to "saw" off the kernels from the cob. You might then sauté the corn in a teaspoon of olive oil with some chopped onion, green pepper, and mushrooms. Add a few egg whites—now that sounds familiar, doesn't it?

Some fast-food restaurants, such as El Pollo Loco and even some of the fried-chicken franchises, sell corn. It is usually dripping in butter, but you can dry off the butter using a napkin or paper towel. This makes the corn healthier and lower in calories.

A tasty variation on corn on the cob: After you wash the ears of corn, soak a paper towel in a little olive oil. Rub down the ears of corn with this oily towel. Next, wrap the ears of corn in aluminum foil and throw them on the barbecue. They need to cook for about 15 minutes, and you need to roll the ears three or four times during that 15 minutes so they won't overcook on any one side.

If you like to eat corn with a fork or spoon instead of off the cob, you can scrape off the kernels from a couple of cooked ears. If you are really into eating slowly, you might try eating this corn with chopsticks! (According to Charles Orben, the "Chinese-food diet" has proved successful in many cases of overweight. On this diet you can eat all you want—with one chopstick.)

Meals on Corn Day

Remember that you can have up to 12 ears of corn on Corn Day. This should be spread out over the entire day. Just as you ate a cup of rice six times a day on Rice Day, you can eat two ears of corn six times on Corn Day. Or you could eat only one ear of corn at a time and have more frequent meals.

Chew Your Corn Well!

You must chew the corn well. You will be able to judge how well you are chewing the corn by looking at your stool the day after Corn Day. If you see large amounts of undigested corn in the stool, this means you haven't chewed well enough; this suggests that you should pay more attention to your chewing at all meals, not only on Corn Day.

According to Herman Aihara, a respected macrobiotics teacher, "chewing well is returning to God." Aihara says that the ancient Japanese had the same idea: *kamu* in Japanese means "to chew," and "*kami*" means "God."

You can see that Corn Day is a very special day. Corn is very satisfying and fulfilling, and it's one of the tastiest foods I know. Enjoy your Corn Day!

Recipe for Corn Day

Corn on the Cob

Basic for any amount of servings. To steam: Steam corn for 5 minutes in a steamer. To boil: Bring water to a rolling boil and carefully place the corn into the pot. Let the water return to a full boil. Cook for 5–7 minutes. To microwave: Microwave corn 4–5 minutes on high; time will vary according to your microwave. Serve with lemon wedges, imitation butter sprinkles, or plain.

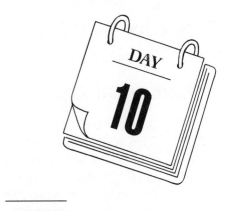

JUICE DAY

Juice Day is best undertaken following one of the heavier days such as Pasta, Corn, Rice, Potato, or Protein Day. Juice Day gives the digestive system a chance to rest, to take a day off, and especially a chance to purify.

Fresh fruit and vegetable juices, especially when squeezed at home with your own juicer, provide the body with great quantities of nutrients. Juice quenches thirst in a satisfying and healthful way and supplies vital energy to the body.

Fruit Juice for Breakfast, Vegetable Juice for Lunch and Dinner

I recommend that you have fruit juice for breakfast and then vegetable juices for lunch and dinner. If fresh vegetable juices are not available, you can use fruit juices throughout the day. Most health-food stores have either fresh-squeezed or bottled vegetable juices. Although fresh vegetable and fruit juices are best, it is certainly possible to use the juices available in any supermarket or health-food store.

Begin the day with an eight-ounce glass of unsweetened orange juice, apple juice, or pineapple juice for breakfast. Any fruit juice is acceptable. If you find the juice too concentrated for your taste, you can dilute it with water. In *midmorning*, if you'd like a snack, you can have six ounces of unsweetened grapefruit juice. For lunch you should have eight ounces of carrot juice if available, or a juice mixture made from green vegetables. No-salt-added tomato juice or no-salt-added V8 juice is also a good choice. In midafternoon you can again have six ounces of grapefruit juice. For dinner drink vegetable juice if it's available; if not, you can choose from grapefruit, orange, or some other fruit juice. An evening snack of grapefruit juice is again acceptable.

How Much Juice to Drink

On Juice Day you can follow the above guidelines for fresh juice or you can have *up to three quarts of store-bought juice per day*, divided as follows: you can have a total of one quart of orange juice and/or unsweetened grapefruit juice. You could mix and have a half quart of orange juice and a half quart of grapefruit juice, or any combination that you wish totaling one quart. The other two quarts of juice can be divided between Hunt's no-salt-added tomato juice, no-salt-added V8 juice, Ocean Spray Low-Calorie Cranberry Juice Cocktail, or Ocean Spray Low-Calorie CranRaspberry Juice Cocktail. Or it can be all or part freshly squeezed fruit or vegetable juice.

One way of supplementing your daily intake of calcium on Juice Day is to use Citrus Hill orange juice and grapefruit juice with added calcium. When you consume a quart of calcium-added juice, you will get your full measure of calcium intake on Juice Day. Several other companies also make calcium-fortified orange juice.

Drink Small Amounts

The best approach is to drink small amounts of juice frequently throughout Juice Day. We are talking about a lot of juice: *up to 12 eight-ounce glasses* as long as you divide it the way that I've outlined above. You don't have to drink that much juice on Juice Day. You can drink less and still derive all of the benefits of the 1-Day-at-a-Time diet.

If you want to put a little fresh lemon juice in the no-salt-added V8 or tomato juice, that's acceptable. You can even add a little bit of pepper or a dash of Tabasco if you wish.

One last word of advice for Juice Day: Don't gulp down your juice too quickly; let it mix with the saliva in your mouth. Sip and savor it like a fine wine.

A Word of Caution on Juice Day

Some people are allergic to citrus fruits. If you are one of these people, you need to substitute other juices for the orange and grapefruit juices recommended on Juice Day. If you were not previously aware of being allergic to citrus fruit but find you have an oversensitivity or some reaction during or immediately after Juice Day, you will need to make substitutions.

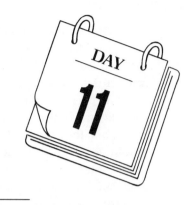

MIX AND MATCH DAY

Mix and Match Day is a preview of the Lifestyle phase, or maintenance diet. The number of ways to mix and match on the 1-Day-at-a-Time diet are unlimited, and I am sure you will be able to think of other ways beyond what I mention here.

I mentioned one mix and match earlier when I told you of the lady who enjoyed the egg-white omelettes so much that she ate them with huge amounts of vegetables throughout the day. She averaged about one pound of weight loss per day while she was eating this way (see page 66).

Meals on Mix and Match Day

How about fruit for breakfast, soup and salad for lunch, a baked potato in the middle of the afternoon, and a broiled defatted, skinned chicken breast with a huge salad and plenty of cooked vegetables for dinner? Eat leftover cooked vegetables for your snack between dinner and bedtime.

Or you could have your egg-white omelette for breakfast (see page 65), a salad and a baked potato with imitation butter flavoring for lunch, a piece of fruit in midmorning and midafternoon, and rice and veggies for dinner. Again, eat the extra cooked vegetables for your snack between dinner and bedtime. Try a liquid protein formula, such as Slim-Fast, for breakfast, a piece of fruit in midmorning, vegetable soup and an ear of corn for lunch, raw vegetables in the afternoon, Pasta Primavera for dinner (see pages 93 and 253), and a five-ounce serving of nonfat frozen yogurt as your evening snack.

As you can see, the opportunities to mix and match the ingredients of the Jump-Start diet for healthful eating are virtually unlimited. I hope by now you are starting to get the picture that the components of the 1-Day-at-a-Time diet are healthy foods, and that when these healthy foods are combined in an intelligent fashion, the diet becomes a wonderfully delicious, healthy, nutritious, low-calorie blessing. You can eat this way every day for the rest of your life; not only will you achieve and maintain your ideal body weight, but you will also be healthy and realize the other benefits of the 1-Day-at-a-Time diet listed in the introduction to this book.

Here's what one of my seminar participants said about Mix and Match Day: "What I have been doing is mixing all the things that you said you could do after you have reached your goal. I find that I could eat that way the rest of my life and I'm still losing three pounds a week. I just pay attention one day at a time."

Recipes for Mix and Match Day

The recipes that follow are only a small example of the many ways to mix and match the components of the 1-Day-at-a-Time diet. Familiarize yourself with the recipes in the recipe section of this book (see page 161) because there are many other recipes that can be used on Mix and Match Day.

Spaghetti Squash Salad

*½ cup cooked spaghetti squash

1 cup diced cooked chicken breast, skinned, all visible fat removed

½ cup thinly sliced celery

½ cup plain nonfat yogurt

Juice of 1 lemon

1 tablespoon pimiento

1 teaspoon vinegar

¼ teaspoon Italian herb seasoning

Cherry tomatoes

Green pepper strips

Combine all ingredients except tomatoes and green pepper; toss lightly with two forks. Adjust seasoning to taste. Chill before serving. Garnish with halved cherry tomatoes and green pepper strips. Serve over a bed of greens. Yields 4–6 servings.

* See basic cooking instructions, page 245.

Tossed Salad with Tuna

1 6½-oz. can water-packed solid white albacore tuna, drained

4 cups mixed salad greens

1 cup sliced green onions

1 green pepper, cut in sticks

½ cup sliced radishes

1 cucumber, cut in sticks

2 carrots, cut in sticks

Cherry tomatoes or tomato wedges

Combine all ingredients except tomatoes in a large bowl; toss. Garnish with cherry tomatoes or tomato wedges. Serve with lemon juice, vinegar, or your favorite no-oil dressing. Yields 4 servings.

Vegetable and Brown Rice Salad

1 cup fresh chop suey vegetables

⅓ cup sliced mushrooms

2 green onions, sliced

1 teaspoon no-oil Italian dressing

½ teaspoon Tamari sauce

⅛ teaspoon dry mustard

⅛ teaspoon ground ginger

1 cup cooked brown rice

Combine all ingredients except rice. Chill and serve over the rice. Yields 2 servings.

Summer Garden Antipasto

1 10-oz. package frozen asparagus spears, or ¾ lb. fresh asparagus

2 cups sliced cucumbers

2 cups sliced mushrooms

1 cup no-oil Italian dressing

1 6½-oz. can water-packed white albacore tuna

Crisp salad greens

2 cups cherry tomatoes

Cook asparagus in ½ cup water until barely tender; drain. Combine cucumbers, mushrooms, and asparagus in a 3-quart glass baking dish with a cover. Pour Italian dressing over the vegetables. Cover and refrigerate at least 1 hour. Drain tuna and remove bottom lid of can so you can push the tuna out in one piece. Place tuna in center of a large serving dish lined with crisp salad greens. Remove vegetables from the dressing, reserving the dressing. Arrange the marinated vegetables and cherry tomatoes around the tuna. Pour dressing over the arrangement. Yields 8 servings.

Stuffed Tomatoes

  2 medium tomatoes
  ½ cup diced cooked chicken breast, skinned, all visible fat removed
  1 tablespoon chopped green onion
  1 rib celery, chopped
  1 teaspoon chopped green pepper
  3 teaspoons no-oil Italian dressing
  1 teaspoon picante sauce (mild)
  ⅛ teaspoon white pepper
     Dash of ground thyme

Hollow out the tomatoes. Chop the flesh and reserve the hollowed-out shells. Lightly toss together chopped tomatoes and all other ingredients. Fill tomato shells with the mixture. Serve on crisp lettuce leaves. Yields 2 servings.

Mushroom Rice Pilaf

½ lb. mushrooms, sliced

½ cup chopped green onions, tops only

2 tablespoons water

2 cups chicken or beef broth, or no-salt-added tomato juice

1 cup uncooked brown rice

Sauté mushrooms and onions in 2 tablespoons water until tender. Add broth and bring to a boil. Place rice in a 2-quart casserole dish and pour the mixture over the rice. Stir. Cover and bake at 350°F. for 1 hour. Yields 6 servings.

Stir-Fried Rice

3 egg whites

3 tablespoons soy sauce

¼ teaspoon ground ginger

⅛ teaspoon garlic powder

3 tablespoons chicken stock or water

1 cup frozen peas, partially thawed

½ cup sliced mushrooms

3 cups cooked brown rice

¼ cup chopped green onions

Green pepper strips

Carrot strips

Lightly beat egg whites, soy sauce, ginger, and garlic powder. Heat 1 tablespoon of chicken stock or water in a nonstick skillet or wok. Add peas and mushrooms.

Stir-fry for 2 minutes. Remove from pan. Add remaining liquid to the pan and heat. Add rice and onions. Stir-fry for 4–6 minutes. Add vegetables and egg mixture. Cook and stir until eggs are set. Garnish with green pepper and carrot strips. Yields 4 servings.

Vegetable Rice Pilaf

1 cup uncooked brown rice

2 cups chicken broth

1 medium onion, chopped

1 small green pepper, cut into thin strips

1 large tomato, diced

2 tablespoons chopped fresh parsley

Combine the rice, chicken broth, and onion in a 1½-quart saucepan. Bring to a boil. Reduce heat. Cover and simmer for 1 hour. Make sure all of the liquid has been absorbed. Stir in green pepper, tomato, and parsley. Heat through. Yields 6–8 servings.

Stir-Fried Vegetables with Brown Rice

½ lb. broccoli

Juice of 1 lemon

3–4 tablespoons chicken stock

1 medium onion, cut in thin vertical slices, then separated into strips

2 ribs celery, thinly sliced

½ small green pepper, chopped

1 cup fresh or frozen corn kernels, thawed

1 cup fresh or frozen cut green beans, thawed

1 teaspoon crushed oregano
White pepper to taste
2 cups cooked brown rice

Cut flowerets from broccoli stem. Place flowerets in 3 cups of water to which lemon juice has been added. Set aside and allow to soak. Peel broccoli stems, then cut into 1-inch slices, then slice again vertically. Heat the chicken stock in a large nonstick skillet over medium heat. Add onion strips, broccoli stem slices, celery, and green pepper. Stir-fry until crisp, about 3 minutes. Drain broccoli flowerets. Add to the onion mixture. Stir in corn, green beans, oregano, and pepper. Stir-fry for 2 minutes or until corn and broccoli flowerets are crispy-tender. Add rice. Stir-fry until hot, about 2 minutes. Yields 4–6 servings.

Steamed Oriental Vegetables and Brown Rice

1¾ cups sliced fresh mushrooms
1½ cups thinly sliced Chinese cabbage
1½ cups diagonally sliced celery
 3 carrots, cut into matchsticks
 2 large onions, thinly sliced
 1 large green pepper, thinly sliced
 1 8-oz. can water chestnuts, drained and sliced
 ½ cup sliced bamboo shoots
 ¼ cup chicken broth
 ¾ cup fresh snow peas
 3 cups bean sprouts
 1 8-oz. can unsweetened pineapple chunks

Combine all vegetables except snow peas and bean sprouts in a large steamer or wok. Add the chicken broth. Cover and steam 4–5 minutes. Add snow peas, bean sprouts, and pineapple. Continue cooking for about 3–4 minutes. Mix thoroughly. If desired, sprinkle with low-sodium soy sauce diluted with equal amount of water. Serve over hot brown rice or Chow Mein Noodles (see recipe on page 232). Yields 6–8 servings.

Pasta Primavera

*1   cone sapsago cheese
4   medium-size carrots, cut in 1-inch pieces
1   lb. broccoli, cut into bite-size pieces
2   medium zucchini, cut in 1-inch pieces
½   lb. spaghetti or corn pasta
1   cup chicken broth
3   teaspoons potato starch or cornstarch
2   cloves garlic, minced
1   lb. cherry tomatoes, halved
2   tablespoons water
1   teaspoon crushed basil
½   lb. mushrooms, sliced
1   10-oz. package frozen peas, slightly thawed
¾   cup chopped parsley

Grate sapsago cheese in a food processor and set aside.

Steam carrots, broccoli, and zucchini until crispy-tender. Put in a large bowl and set aside.

Cook spaghetti al dente. Drain and set aside.

Combine chicken broth and potato starch or corn-

---

* Sapsago cheese is a hard, nonfat cheese that comes in the shape of a small cone. If unavailable, use a *very small* amount of Romano or Parmesan cheese.

starch. Stir until smooth. Bring to a boil, then reduce heat to simmer. Cook and stir until thickened. Set aside.

Sauté garlic and tomatoes in a large nonstick skillet with 2 tablespoons water for 2 minutes. Stir in basil and mushrooms. Cook 2 more minutes. Stir in peas and parsley. Cook 1 more minute. Add to steamed vegetables in the bowl.

In the large nonstick skillet, add cooked spaghetti to the thickened chicken broth mixture and toss to coat. Stir in the vegetables. Heat slowly until hot. Sprinkle the cheese lightly over the Pasta Primavera. Yields 6 servings.

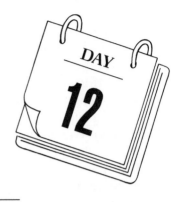

LIQUID PROTEIN DAY

Liquid Protein Day is included in Jump-Start to emphasize the utility of this wonderful tool in your dieting lifestyle. When I say "liquid protein" I mean products such as Slim-Fast, Twinfast, and Carnation Instant Breakfast. When prepared with skim or nonfat milk, these diet shakes provide a well-balanced, highly nutritious meal with about 200 calories and an extremely low fat and cholesterol count.

There are a wide variety of flavors available in these products, and I find them all quite tasty. One trick for making a tastier drink is to pour skim milk into an ice tray and freeze it. Then when you prepare the drink, add about half liquid skim milk and half frozen skim-milk ice cubes to the blender. This will make it a creamier, "milkshakier" drink and to my taste buds a tastier one. You can experiment and try all the flavors and find the ones that are most pleasing to you.

Slim-Fast also makes a product called Ultra Slim-Fast, which has more fiber than regular Slim-Fast. I personally prefer the regular version, but you can experiment with a can of Ultra Slim-Fast and see if this extra fiber is useful to you. Some people will find that it creates excessive gas.

Twinfast (only available in health-food stores) has the advantage that it can be made with water (ice cubes). This yields a delicious meal for only 80 calories.

In my experience, the medically supervised programs that utilize liquid diets such as Optifast and Medifast are less than satisfactory. People who lose their weight exclusively on these liquid diets almost always gain it back. The difficulty with this kind of diet is that you never learn how to eat in a healthy fashion on a day-to-day basis—as you would, for example, if you utilized the principles outlined in the Lifestyle phase of the 1-Day-at-a-Time diet.

Having said all this, I again emphasize that liquid formulas such as Slim-Fast and Twinfast are exceptionally useful as an *adjunct* to any weight-loss program.

Meals on Liquid Protein Day

Liquid Protein Day is, in effect, a Mix and Match Day. On this day, you'll use two diet shakes in place of two meals. It usually works best to have a diet shake for breakfast and lunch and eat a nutritious meal for dinner.

Dinner might be a broiled chicken breast that has been skinned and defatted, a raw vegetable salad, and cooked vegetables. Another option is a bowl of Edythe's Fresh Vegetable Soup (see pages 62 and 196), and a baked potato *or* an ear of corn.

On Liquid Protein Day you can have unlimited amounts of raw vegetables—such as carrots, zucchini, cucumber, and celery—between meals. Leftover cooked vegetables or another cup of vegetable soup will serve as your snack between dinner and bedtime.

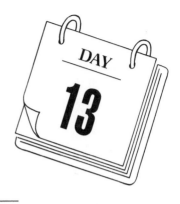

REPEAT YOUR FAVORITE DAY

The Repeat Your Favorite Day on the 1-Day-at-a-Time diet plan is a day you will use repeatedly for the rest of your life. It's the day you go back to whenever you've slipped off your diet. If you go to a party, or out to dinner, or to someone's house, or you let your self-control down for a few minutes and find that you've eaten things you know you shouldn't have, it doesn't mean that you have spoiled all the good work you have done up until then. It just means that you stepped off the path. What do you do when you step off the path? You get back on the path, you take it not only one day at a time but one step at a time. You must acknowledge that to be human is to be frail and to be frail is to have weakness.

If you binge or go off the diet, don't get caught up in self-blame. Don't think, "There goes my diet—I have ruined it all." The fact of the matter is, it just isn't true. All you have to do is get back on the path, and the way you do that is by returning to your favorite day on the 1-Day-at-a-

97

Time diet, the day that you most enjoyed and had fun with. Then do another day or two of your favorite days before returning to the Mix and Match or the Lifestyle phase, and you will find that you'll hardly miss a step on your path to health, happiness, self-esteem, and slimness.

Lifestyle

Guide to Weight Loss and Health Maintenance

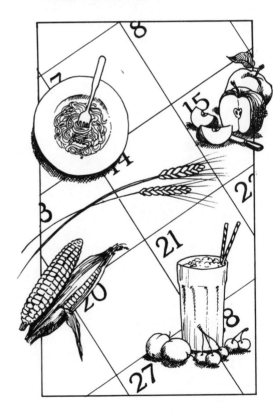

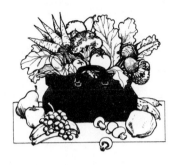

In Jump-Start, you learned a technique for rapid weight loss using healthy foods one day at a time. In Lifestyle, you will learn the principles of healthy eating to continue your weight loss and to maximize your chances of reducing your risk of heart disease, certain cancers, diabetes, constipation, and hypertension. The principles for healthy eating and exercise are contained in the 15 sections that comprise the Lifestyle phase.

Information on how to incorporate these principles into your day-to-day eating is contained in the Master Plan immediately following the Lifestyle principles (see page 151). Recipes for helping you implement this Master Plan are found on page 161.

UNDERSTANDING FATS AND CHOLESTEROL

My old friend and teacher Nathan Pritikin based his nutritional program on the elimination of all fats from the diet. To a large degree the success of the Pritikin program is directly related to a person's ability to accomplish this end. In fact, Pritikin was preoccupied with the elimination of fats from the diet.

Since Pritikin's pioneering work in the 1970s, scientists have recognized that some fats in limited quantities can be beneficial—namely, certain vegetable oils such as olive oil and fish oils. We'll talk more about them in a moment.

The most important secret I have learned about weight loss and maintaining weight loss is that *the total amount of fat in your diet must be held to an absolute minimum.* The reason for this is that fats have more concentrated calories than do carbohydrates or protein, so that one gram of fat has nine calories, whereas one gram of carbohydrate or protein has only four calories. Therefore, any successful approach to weight loss must eliminate as much fat as possible. *If you don't eat fat, you can burn the fat that you already have stored in your body,* and that means *you will lose weight.*

It is not always easy to eliminate fats because they are often hidden, and unless you know what foods are high in fat you would not necessarily restrict that food. For example, all nuts (with the exception of chestnuts) are loaded with fat. Cheese, butter, and whole milk all have more than 50 percent of their calories in fat. Mayonnaise, avocado, and coconut are loaded with fat. Cream soups, nondairy creamers, and whipped-cream substitutes are all high in fat content. These are foods that must be eliminated from the diet in order to have a successful weight-loss and weight-maintenance program.

Just as olive oil and fish oils are beneficial, certain fats are harmful. Excessive amounts of saturated fats and cholesterol are abundant in animal foods and dairy products. Red meat and butter are harmful because they raise the cholesterol level of the blood. The higher the blood cholesterol level, the more likely that the cholesterol will be deposited in the arteries; when this occurs the result is heart attack, stroke, and/or death.

Another term for saturated fat is "hydrogenated fat"; therefore you should read the labels on products you buy in the supermarket. If you see that one of the ingredients is "partially hydrogenated oil," avoid the product if possible. Essentially all fried foods in fast-food restaurants are fried in hydrogenated fats. Coconut oil, a major ingredient in many nondairy creamers, is hydrogenated and should be eliminated from everyone's diet.

Fats and Cancer

In studying population groups, doctors have discovered that the highest incidence of colon cancer occurs in countries with the highest meat consumption—for example, the

United States, Canada, Scotland, and New Zealand. In Japan, where there is less fat intake, bowel cancer occurs less than one-third as frequently as in the United States. It has been shown that when Japanese people emigrate to the United States and adopt a modern American diet with emphasis on meat and dairy products, they show the same colon cancer statistics as Americans.

Overconsumption of fat and cholesterol has been shown to contribute to other cancers as well. According to the National Cancer Institute, fats accelerate the growth of breast tumors. Dr. Ernst Wynder of the American Health Foundation has done research confirming this relationship between breast cancer and fat intake.

Fats and Heart Disease

Coronary heart disease and atherosclerosis in all of its forms currently account for more than one-half of all deaths in the United States. Over one million Americans will have heart attacks this year. One out of four Americans suffers from some form of cardiovascular disease. The underlying cause of the vast majority of heart attacks is cholesterol-laden fatty deposits in the blood vessels. Atherosclerosis results in narrowing of the arteries, which restricts the supply of oxygen to the affected tissues. Due to the enormous amount of fats consumed in the United States, nearly *half* of all males in their early twenties already have evidence of atherosclerosis.

Dr. Ancel Keys and his colleagues, heart researchers at the University of Minnesota, have found that in Scandinavian countries—where a high percentage of total calories comes from saturated fats—rates of death from cardiovascular disease are much higher than in Mediterranean countries, such as Greece and Italy, where most of the fat consumed is unsaturated (olive oil). Recent studies have shown that when the high-fat Scandinavian diet was changed to a healthier, low-fat diet, there was a decreased incidence of heart disease.

Many other studies throughout the world have confirmed the fact that it is possible to control and reverse the process of atherosclerosis through a change in diet—namely, by the elimination of saturated fats and cholesterol. The huge amount of research and medical findings on the causes of heart disease has led health organizations throughout the world to urge people to decrease consumption of fat and cholesterol. *The single most important dietary change that most Americans could make would be to decrease or eliminate saturated fats and cholesterol from their diets.*

In fact, in June 1987 there was an article published in the *Journal of the American Medical Association* by Dr. David Blankenhorn of the University of Southern California, Los Angeles. This study proved for the first time that lowering serum cholesterol results in a reversal of obstruction in the coronary arteries in human beings. The importance of this study is that it establishes *as fact* that by lowering cholesterol we can clean out the arteries that bring blood to our hearts, and thereby reduce our risk of heart attack.

The Olive Oil Story

It has been known for many years that there are fewer heart attacks than would be expected in several of the Mediterranean countries, as noted earlier. This reduction in the risk of heart attack was in some regard independent of the level of serum cholesterol. That is, for any given level of serum cholesterol, people in the United States and Western Europe were having more heart attacks than people in the Mediterranean countries with the same level of cholesterol in their blood.

An explanation for this phenomenon was sought. It was largely due to the research of Dr. Scott Grundy at the University of Texas Health Sciences Center in Dallas that we learned the mechanism of how olive oil seems to protect against heart attack. Not only is the "bad" cholesterol (LDL) lowered, but the "good" cholesterol (HDL) is raised when the diet is rich in olive oil. Olive oil also seems to create some protection against clotting, which plays a role with cholesterol in the formation of artery blockages.

The Fish Oil Story

Credit for unraveling the fish oil mystery goes to Dr. William Connor at the Oregon Health Sciences University located in Portland.

Just as it was noted that people in certain Mediterranean countries are protected against heart disease, it was also known for many years that the Eskimos, who ate a high-fat diet, seldom had heart attacks. Doctors suspected that there was something very special about those fish oils the Eskimos were eating in large quantities. Eskimos are not skinny—they have a lot of fat on their bones to keep them warm in the freezing winters—but they have few heart attacks. We do want to keep sight of the fact that our objective is to be healthy and lean, although there is a lesson to be learned from the Eskimos. The fats that are present in the fish—the fish oils—give protection against clotting and in this way protect against artery blockage.

The best fish to eat are those that come from cold, clean waters, namely around Alaska, Newfoundland, Greenland, and the North Sea. Alaskan salmon is a good example of a healthy fish. As of this writing there has been no indication of contamination of the fish population around the waters of the 1989 Exxon Valdez oil spill. However, we must keep a close watch for signs of contamination in the future. Fishes that are scavengers, such as shark, are not to be eaten on a regular basis because all of the pollutants, such as mercury and DDT, are more concentrated the higher up the food chain you go. That means that whatever pollutants are eaten by the smaller fish are incorporated into the larger scavenger fish and multiplied by the number of smaller fish the larger fish (like the shark) have eaten. These pollutants are transferred to your body when you consume those fish.

One of the best fish of all to eat is sardines. The little sardines do not eat other fishes. They eat plankton from the ocean, and the sardine oil itself seems to be one of the most protective fish oils available. Most cans of sardines contain about 200 calories of oil. Drain as much of the oil from the sardines as possible to minimize calories. Best of all, buy your sardines packed in sild sardine oil or olive oil.

Other Oils

In addition to fish oils and olive oil, certain other oils are healthy and sometimes useful in an overall nutrition program.

Canola oil, which is produced from rapeseed, has many characteristics in common with olive oil and in addition has about 10 percent of its fat in the same form as fish oil. Canola oil is available in health-food stores from a company called Spectrum and in supermarkets as Puritan oil (produced by Procter and Gamble). The flavor of canola oil is milder than olive oil, and it can be mixed with olive oil to balance the flavor for those of you who find olive oil too strong.

Another healthy oil is flaxseed oil. Flaxseed oil is essentially the vegetable equivalent of fish oil. It's a very delicate oil and is best stored in the refrigerator. It is so delicate that it cannot be used for frying. Once you reach your ideal weight and want to add small amounts of oil to your salad dressing, flaxseed oil will make a tasty and healthy variation.

How does all this information translate into what you can do on a day-to-day basis to stay healthy as well as slim? The answer is simple: *Make fish the major source of animal protein in your diet*. In addition, whenever you use a cooking oil, whether it is to sauté or to make a salad dressing or to cook a muffin, make olive oil your first choice. Canola and flaxseed are a close second.

Avoid Fatty Foods!

By now it should be obvious that consumption of fatty foods will damage your body and create havoc with your weight. Fats suffocate your tissues by depriving them of oxygen; they raise cholesterol levels in the blood; and they impede the digestion of carbohydrates, causing weight gain and fostering diabetes. There is yet another problem with consuming fatty foods: pesticides and other chemical pollutants tend to be stored in animal fat cells, so when you eat fatty animal products you may be ingesting doses of poison. You can get all the fat you need by eating vegetables and grains. After you have completed Jump-Start, and as you begin to approach your ideal weight, you can add small amounts of olive oil, canola oil, and flaxseed oil to your diet. Since worldwide studies have proven that a low-fat diet will significantly reduce your chances of having a heart attack, and since we know that fats and saturated oils play a role in cancer and will fatten you up and shorten your life, why not follow this formerly fat doctor's advice and eat small amounts of healthy fats and *eliminate saturated fats and oils from your diet.*

Eggs

It's funny sometimes how as we get older and smarter we find that we know less and less. Twenty years ago I thought I knew the answer to whether eggs are healthy or not. It seemed simple enough: Each egg yolk contains somewhere in the neighborhood of 250 milligrams of cholesterol. The more cholesterol we eat, the more cholesterol the liver has to deal with and the more likely we are to build up cholesterol deposits in our arteries. There is no cholesterol (or fat) in egg whites.

But eggs aren't always as simple as they seem. Several studies have been done in which healthy people ate large numbers of eggs on a daily basis for a prolonged period of time without any rise in their blood cholesterol level. This in itself does not insure that the cholesterol in eggs does not contribute to cholesterol deposits in the arteries. There are other examples of this phenomenon. The Masai, a tribe in Africa that eats a diet high in animal fat and cholesterol, has low blood cholesterol on the average and yet they have extensive atherosclerosis.

There is a whole body of literature written on how the lecithin in egg yolks helps with their metabolism and assimilation so as to prevent the cholesterol from being deposited in the arteries. To the best of my knowledge, there is no real evidence to support this line of reasoning.

It may be that the way the egg is prepared has something to do with the quality of the cholesterol and how it is handled by the body. Several studies have shown that oxidized cholesterol—that is, cholesterol that is subjected to high levels of heat—is handled differently in the body. This may mean that eggs that are poached, soft-boiled, or hard-boiled are more healthful than fried eggs.

At this time it is impossible to answer the question as to whether egg yolks are healthy or not. So, what is my recommendation? Well, if you eat eggs and they are not healthy, you have done yourself a disservice; if you do not eat eggs and they are healthy, you will have done yourself much less of a disservice. Until all the answers are in, you should limit your egg intake to *no more than two egg yolks a week* and whenever possible poach, or soft or hard boil the eggs instead of frying. Frying egg whites is just fine.

2

ELIMINATE SUGAR

We have heard a lot about sugar over the years. Everyone from Adele Davis to Nathan Pritikin has cautioned us about the evils of sugar. Is sugar bad, and if so why?

Unfortunately, excessive amounts of sugar play havoc with your metabolism, your weight, and your willpower. Sugar is like a loose cannon. It enters the bloodstream immediately after you ingest it and begins to do its damage to your metabolism from that point onward. The body responds to the sugar rush by pumping out high doses of insulin. This may result in hypoglycemia, or low blood sugar, a few hours later. In addition, the increased levels of insulin may injure the walls of your arteries and make them more vulnerable to deposits of cholesterol and fats.

One of the biggest problems with this sugar-insulin interaction is that the outpouring of insulin drives the blood sugar down and this low blood sugar causes a hunger attack that is like no other. Because sugar is necessary for the brain to survive, the body tends to protect the brain and make sure that the blood sugar levels stay in a healthy range. When you eat large amounts of sugar, the insulin that follows will drive the blood sugar down so that hunger will force you to eat in order to protect your brain cells. It's a vicious cycle that is impossible to break—unless you stop eating sugar. The body needs sugar and the brain must have a continuous supply of sugar—but the way you should get sugar is from complex carbohydrates, not from simple sugars. Simple sugar is concentrated in fruit juices, fruit, honey, molasses, fructose, corn syrup, and malted barley, as well as table sugar.

This roller coaster pattern of sugar intake and out-pouring of insulin, with the resultant low blood sugar and hunger, is also responsible for an emotional roller coaster and rapidly changing moods in many people. Some hyperactive children will "mellow out" when simple sugar is eliminated from their diet.

The most important thing to remember is that you will lessen your chances of attaining your goal of healthful lean-ness as long as you continue to incorporate sugar in your diet.

Fruit Day, Frozen Yogurt Day, and Juice Day

There are three days in the Jump-Start phase of this diet that contain high amounts of simple sugar—Fruit Day, Frozen Yogurt Day, and Juice Day. My experience in using these days is that they are in general well tolerated by most people. If you have a sensitivity to sugar, do not use the Frozen Yogurt Day or the Fruit Day in Jump-Start. Instead, substitute other light days, such as Soup Day, Vegetable Day, or Liquid Protein Day.

Juice Day includes some sugar in the orange juice. My experience has been that Juice Day does not pose a problem with most people who are sensitive to sugar because it has been constructed to stress low-sugar juices such as no-salt-added V8, no-salt-added tomato juice, and low-calorie juice cocktails. If you are concerned about Juice Day having too much sugar, however, substitute one of the other light days of Jump-Start.

In the Lifestyle, or maintenance, phase of this diet you must limit your fruit juices to no more than six ounces of regular juice per day. However, you can have unlimited amounts of no-salt-added tomato and V8 juice cocktail. In order to minimize your simple-sugar intake, you must limit your fruit intake to no more than four fruits per day in the Lifestyle phase.

3

COMPLEX CARBOHYDRATES

Complex carbohydrates are made up of simple sugars that are bound together in such a way that they are digested slowly and enter the bloodstream slowly, like time-released energy. That way they do not result in excessive production of insulin. Complex carbohydrates are found in whole grains such as rice, corn, wheat, barley, and oats. Vegetables are complex carbohydrates that do not contain a lot of calories. Potatoes act as though they are half complex carbohydrate and half simple sugar.

If you eat simple sugars your energy level will be like a roller coaster, rising up and then crashing. With complex carbohydrates your energy will be sustained and balanced throughout the day. Complex carbohydrates are fuel for sustained or endurance exercise. Marathon runners will "carb-up" for days before a race in order to build up the complex carbohydrate (glycogen) stores in their muscles.

Because complex carbohydrates will prevent the insulin-hypoglycemia roller coaster, they will also keep you from getting hungry.

Avoid Eating Bread

You may have noticed that no place else in the book do I suggest eating bread. Bread is made of flour, which is ground wheat—a complex carbohydrate. However, my experience over the years has been that it is very difficult to lose weight and keep it off if you suffer from a sluggish metabolism and eat bread or crackers. It even goes a little further than that: It seems that the majority of people who have a weight problem do substantially better on their diet if they minimize their wheat intake. The only wheat allowed on this diet is in the pasta and in the bran muffins.

Once you have achieved your desired weight you may experiment with small amounts of bread. But be careful. If your weight starts to go back up, bread must be one of the first things you strike out of your diet.

4

EAT MORE VEGETABLES

If you want to remain healthy and slim for the rest of your life you must *eat more vegetables*! The high water content and extremely low calorie content of vegetables will insure that you stay thin and still feel satisfied after meals. Vegetable fibers exert an "anti-blood-fat" effect, reducing elevated cholesterol levels and promoting good digestion and good health. *The more vegetables you eat, the more weight you will lose.*

Abundant medical and scientific evidence shows that more vegetables in your diet can decrease your risk of heart disease and cancer. "Increase the amount of fruits and vegetables in your diet," says the National Cancer Institute. In 1983 the American Cancer society stated, "A greater use of fruits and vegetables can significantly reduce a person's risk of developing cancer."

It has been found that the "cruciferous" vegetables, which include cabbage, broccoli, Brussels sprouts, cauliflower, and turnips, contain substances that stimulate the immune system and help protect against cancer-causing agents.

Most Impressive Weight Loss

The most impressive weight-loss cases I have seen involve patients who eat mostly vegetables and fruits after a lifetime of eating more fatty foods. In the past 10 years I have worked with hundreds of people who have adopted a predominantly vegetarian diet with small amounts of fruit, grains, and protein. Weight losses of *15 to 25 pounds a month* are common among these people, with the added benefit that they never feel hungry or deprived.

One secretary who began this diet over a weekend reported a six-pound weight loss from Friday afternoon to Monday morning! Although this weight loss was mostly water, it was nonetheless inspiring to her. This kind of encouragement is important to maintain a lifestyle change, and this is exactly what you can expect on the 1-Day-at-a-Time diet.

The more vegetables you eat, the more you fill up with fiber and water (and treasures of vitamins, minerals, and enzymes). You won't feel hungry after your meals, and *you won't gain weight!*

You can prepare vegetables in a variety of healthy ways—steam them, boil them, put them in soups, bake them. You can even sauté them in a small amount of olive oil or defatted chicken broth with herbs and seasonings. They will be truly delicious and will satisfy any gourmet palate.

Whenever possible, eat vegetables raw as well as cooked. Raw vegetables retain more of the water-soluble vitamins and minerals. You can also use a microwave to cook crisp and nutritious vegetables. For cooking times, follow the suggestions in the booklet that came with your microwave. Eat as many raw or microwaved vegetables as you wish. You can nibble on vegetables all day long. Choose a variety of colors—red, orange, yellow, green—to make interesting and visually pleasing meals (not just side dishes) of nutritious vegetables.

Contrary to what you may have learned as a child if you were conditioned to hate vegetables, this cornucopia food group can be prepared in wonderful and varied ways to create excellent meals.

Try New Vegetables

Learn about exotic vegetables. Shop for them in ethnic markets and farmers' markets. Try new ones you see in the supermarket. By serving interesting vegetable dishes and vegetable soups combined with different grains, for example, you can shift the emphasis of your family's meals away from meat dishes.

Keep your refrigerator filled with lots of vegetables— not just the traditional "salad vegetables" like different kinds of lettuce, cucumbers, green peppers, carrots, and tomatoes, but also with the makings of hot main vegetable dishes. There are many such dishes among my mother's recipes in this book.

Vegetables contain so many vitamins, minerals, and enzymes, as well as fiber, in relation to their caloric content that you and your family will experience improved health and weight maintenance even if you heed only this one section of the maintenance diet—*eat more vegetables!*

5

FABULOUS FIBER

At age 17 I went on a diet and lost 45 pounds in approximately two months. I didn't really know what I was doing; I just restricted my calories to about 600 per day and exercised like crazy. I paid no attention to fiber, and as a 17-year-old kid I didn't even know what the word *constipation* meant. The constipation that resulted from that low-fiber diet has left me with a hemorrhoid that I still have today.

Over the next 25 years I suffered from an elimination problem. It was not until 1977 when I met Nathan Pritikin and learned about fiber that I was able to solve this problem. In my private practice I see people every day who suffer with a similar problem and I am always amazed that they don't know about fiber, because it seems to me that there is so much written now on the use of fiber to control constipation.

Kinds of Fiber

You can get fiber from many sources: fruit, vegetables, beans, peas, legumes, grains. A very special source of fiber is psyllium husks, which come from the coating of the plant Plantago ovata.

Many people who have good elimination do not have to supplement their diet with extra fiber; they get plenty from fruits, vegetables, and whole grains. People who are on a healthy diet often speak of one of the advantages of this diet as being good elimination. However, others who seem to have a more sluggish colon can eat a "healthy diet" and still have elimination problems. These people need to go out of their way to add a little extra fiber to their diet.

I bet you didn't appreciate that the reason you get gas from beans is that beans are high in fiber. The fiber goes through the intestinal tract and by the time it gets to the colon the bacteria that live in the colon break down the fiber. The bacteria can digest the fiber but we can't; when the bacteria digests the fiber, one of the by-products is gas. Some raw vegetables such as cauliflower and broccoli cause gas in some people. Wheat bran and wheat fiber as well as oat bran and some fruits (prunes) can also cause gas.

How to Add Fiber to Your Diet

Some of you will find that simply by switching from the fatty animal-based protein diet that you have been on, and incorporating more fruits, vegetables, and whole grains into your diet, your elimination will improve. If this is not the case, you could add a teaspoon or two of psyllium husks to your diet each day. This is available in health-food stores as well as in the commercial product Metamucil. If you start using psyllium husks, begin with only one teaspoon per day and gradually increase an additional teaspoon a day every three to five days to make sure you do not get too much psyllium in your diet. An extra advantage of psyllium is that it has been shown to reduce blood cholesterol levels. Be sure to drink an extra glass of water with your psyllium; it will help you feel full. You can use psyllium if it becomes necessary at any time in this diet. In my experience it is rarely necessary to use more than two or three teaspoons of psyllium husks per day, and often one teaspoon is sufficient

Bran Muffin Snack

One of my patients, Christi, has created one of the most wonderful bran muffin recipes I have ever come across. I have included this recipe in the fiber section here for easy reference (see page 122). A bran muffin makes an excellent snack, and many people find that one bran muffin a day is all they need to guarantee perfect regularity. These muffins are really special because they contain both wheat bran and oat bran.

These two brans are each important and play a different and vital role in health. While the wheat bran is important for bulk and colon health, the oat bran may be helpful in reducing serum cholesterol and lowering your risk of heart attack. You should use this special recipe to make your own muffins because it combines the wheat and oat brans in a ratio that will help to optimize your elimination as well as lower your serum cholesterol. The muffins you buy in the store are all too high in fat and/or sugar and have too many calories to be usable on the 1-Day-at-a-Time diet. So if you can't or won't make your own muffins, don't substitute store-bought muffins.

You should at least experiment and make these muffins once. You will find that it is not that hard. You can make double the recipe and freeze half to three-quarters of the muffins to have them ready for another day. You will enjoy these bran muffins as a snack between meals and they will play a useful and healthy role in your Lifestyle or maintenance diet.

Fabulous Fiber Recipe

Christi's Basic Muffin Recipe

1½ cups whole-wheat flour

⅓ cup oat bran

⅓ cup wheat bran

3 tablespoons nonfat dry milk powder

*2 teaspoons Rumsford baking powder

½ teaspoon freshly grated orange peel

2 teaspoons cinnamon

5 egg whites

5 tablespoons honey

3 tablespoons oil (canola, olive, or safflower)

2 teaspoons vanilla extract (don't use imitation vanilla flavoring)

Variations (choose one):

1 cup shredded carrots

1 cup shredded zucchini

1 cup mashed bananas

1 cup chopped berries or cherries

1 cup blueberries, fresh or frozen

Preheat oven to 350°F. Stir together the first seven ingredients in a large bowl. Puree remaining ingredients in blender or use hand mixer (this is a very important step). Add pureed liquid to dry mixture and stir well

---

* Rumsford baking powder is lower in sodium than other brands and contains no aluminum sulfate.

(DO NOT BEAT). The mixture will be thick like a cookie dough. Mix in choice of variation until well distributed. By hand, divide the dough into 12 portions and put into paper-lined muffin cups. Bake at 350°F. for about 17 minutes or until top begins to darken and center springs back when lightly pressed. Yields 12 muffins.

6

EAT MODERATE AMOUNTS OF PROTEIN

If you don't eat enough protein you will break down your body's own protein. Even though you lose weight, it will be muscle and organ mass that you lose rather than fatty tissue. Extended diets consisting of only vegetables, or water or juice fasts for long periods of time, result in organ tissue breakdown and are dangerous. It is possible to be a vegetarian and get all the protein you need. I remember a few years ago seeing the cover of a magazine, *Vegetarian Times*, showing a weightlifter with huge muscles. Inside he explained how he was able to build his muscles on a pure vegetarian diet. In order to do that you need to know what you are doing and how to insure that you get all the amino acids you need. Advice on how to become a pure vegetarian is beyond the scope of this book.

It is my recommendation that you eat small amounts of healthful animal protein, such as fish; defatted, skinned breast of chicken and turkey; egg whites; nonfat or skim milk; and liquid protein supplements such as Slim-Fast or

Twinfast. When a healthy diet of fruits, vegetables, and whole grains is supplemented with moderate amounts of these proteins, you get all the protein you need without excessive amounts of cholesterol, which is found only in animal tissues. Egg whites and skim milk are good sources of cholesterol-free, no-fat protein.

If you eat too much protein you run the risk of consuming excessive fat and cholesterol. In addition, if you eat excessive amounts of protein, you will lose calcium from your bones. Protein is made up of amino acids. These acids need to be balanced or buffered by calcium salts. In order to do this, the body takes calcium out of the bones and excretes it in the urine. Excessive protein intake thus will result in weak bones. Excessive means more than 90 grams of protein per day.

How to Get All the Healthy Protein You Need

Do not eat more than eight ounces of animal flesh per day. This includes fish, breast of chicken and turkey, and extra-lean beef such as flank steak. You may also have up to four glasses of nonfat/skim milk per day, up to four egg whites per day, and up to eight ounces of nonfat yogurt. There is no cheese other than nonfat cottage cheese or sapsago cheese on this diet because cheese is too high in fat. If you use the liquid protein drinks such as Slim-Fast, you should reduce your animal protein intake proportionally.

7

CONSUME ONLY NONFAT DAIRY PRODUCTS

If you don't eat fat you will be able to burn your body's own fat stores and become thin. One of the major hidden sources of fat in the American diet is dairy products. In terms of percentage of calories, cheese is 70 to 80 percent fat; sour cream the same; whole milk is 54 percent fat; ice cream is better than 70 percent fat; cream is 100 percent fat; butter and margarine are 100 percent fat. So if you want to eliminate animal fat from your diet you have to eat only nonfat dairy products. There is no reason not to: You get all of the nutrition, all of the calcium, all of the protein, and all of the good taste when you eat nonfat dairy products.

Cholesterol is found only in animal products. When the fat is removed from dairy products, the cholesterol, which is soluble in the fat, is also removed; so nonfat milk and nonfat yogurt are not only fat free but are also cholesterol free. They're both excellent sources of protein; a glass of skim or nonfat milk has approximately nine grams of protein and about one-third of your daily requirement of calcium. You get all of the good stuff from the nonfat dairy products and none of the bad stuff.

Cottage cheese, on the other hand, contains protein, but the calcium has been removed in the making of the cottage cheese. Nonfat milk and nonfat yogurt are better choices than nonfat cottage cheese.

Calcium

Dairy products are the best natural source of calcium. If you consume nonfat dairy products you will be getting healthy calcium in your diet. Adults need at least 1,000 milligrams of calcium in their diet each day. If there is a long-term chronic calcium deficiency in the diet, the body will reabsorb calcium from the skeleton and weaken the bones, resulting in osteoporosis. Exercise is also a necessary ingredient to help keep calcium in the bones. In sedentary, inactive people, calcium is reabsorbed from the bones regardless of how much calcium is in the diet. This is also true if protein intake is excessive. More than 90 grams of protein per day will cause an obligatory reabsorption from the bones to buffer the excessive amino acids. So, consuming enough calcium is only one of a series of complicated interactions that are necessary in order to maintain bone integrity. I will tell you more about calcium supplementation in the Vitamin and Mineral Supplements chapter (see page 142).

8

USE SALT WITH CAUTION

When I was an intern under a great deal of stress and working extremely long hours, I stopped one day and took my blood pressure and found it to be elevated—145/95, much too high for a young man. So at that juncture in my life I began to study with a very personal interest causes and treatment of blood pressure elevation. I wasn't very excited about a lifetime of drugs, and so when I learned that restriction of salt can cure high blood pressure in some people, I eliminated salt from my diet. Almost immediately my blood pressure began to fall. When I had an insurance examination seven months later my pressure was 120/70.

Since that time I have continued to be conscious of the amount of salt added to foods that I buy and I have never again used a salt shaker. My pressure has continued to be in the 120/70 range all this time—25 years. The usual pattern for young men with mildly elevated blood pressure, such as I had, is for the problem to steadily progress with age. So salt restriction can definitely make a difference. Not only do you need to eliminate salt from your diet, you also need to eliminate foods that have large quantities of salt or sodium added to them, such as most canned soups.

The most widely prescribed medicines for high blood pressure are diuretics. The only thing a diuretic does is help the kidneys get rid of salt, so many of the people who are taking diuretics for high blood pressure might be able to get by without the diuretic if they eliminated salt from their diet.

In addition, there are some other natural things that can help lower blood pressure, such as supplementing your diet with calcium, magnesium, and potassium. Ask your doctor. *Don't stop your medication without your doctor's knowledge.*

Not Everyone Needs to Eliminate Salt

If your blood pressure normally runs in the 120/70 range or lower and you currently add salt to your food, you should not eliminate salt from your diet, because if you do your blood pressure will go down and could get too low. Because the risk of heart disease is directly related to the level of blood pressure, the lower the blood pressure the better, as long as you don't have symptoms of low blood pressure. The symptoms of low blood pressure are dizziness or light-headedness when rising from a sitting or lying position. As long as there are no such symptoms, it's hard for blood pressure to be too low.

9

EAT LESS AND LIVE LONGER

Roy L. Walford, M.D., has been a professor of pathology at the UCLA School of Medicine since 1966. He has spent his professional career as a researcher in pursuit of ways of prolonging life-span. Dr. Walford has looked at essentially every possible mechanism for slowing the aging process, extending life, and maintaining a healthy and active mind and body.

He has found that some drugs and supplements are beneficial. However, there is one mechanism that most consistently increased the life-span in his research on animals. It is not uncommon for him to increase longevity in research animals by 30 to 50 percent. This one mechanism that consistently prolongs life is *the eating of fewer calories*.

The induction of leanness through underfeeding, when combined with adequate levels of vitamin and mineral supplements, not only prolongs life, but the added years are full of health and vigor.

The secret is eating fewer calories and maintaining your weight at a healthy lean level. And that's exactly what the 1-Day-at-a-Time diet teaches you to do.

PRINCIPLE

10

FINESSING FAST FOODS AND RESTAURANTS

The best place to conduct your 1-Day-at-a-Time diet is at home. But sometimes you are out and hungry, and sometimes for social reasons you find yourself in a restaurant. This chapter will help you make intelligent decisions when you find yourself in these situations.

What to Order

You can get a fine vegetable salad at any restaurant. You can even get them to make you a double- or triple-size salad. If you haven't brought your own nonfat or calorie-reduced salad dressing, you can always use lemon juice or vinegar. Or order dressing on the side; put one or two teaspoons of the house dressing on your salad, then dress the rest of the salad with lemon juice or vinegar in order to minimize calories.

Order a chicken breast or piece of fish grilled dry; be sure to tell the waiter no added butter. If the chicken comes with the skin on, remove the skin. Many restaurants will prepare a large platter of steamed vegetables. If you order a baked potato, be sure to get it plain. If you plan ahead you can carry imitation butter sprinkle (Molly McButter, Best o' Butter, Butter Buds, Instead of Butter) with you to put on the baked potato. For dessert you can have a piece of fresh fruit.

You can order this meal or a variation of it at most restaurants.

Fast-Food Restaurants

Wendy's has a salad bar that is out of this world. They even have a reduced-calorie dressing available. They also sell baked potatoes, and you can get one plain. There is also pasta on the salad bar, but pass on the pasta if you order the baked potato, and vice versa. Pass the greasy stuff by. Steak houses such as The Sizzler and Steak and Ale have wonderful salad bars and baked potatoes available. At the salad bar, choose the fresh vegetables and stay away from the potato salad and mayonnaise-ladden coleslaw. Say no to the toast and ask for plenty of lemons for salad dressing, or bring your own dressing. Chili's has a delicious salad with grilled chicken breast added. Again, use a few tea-spoons of the house dressing, then lots of lemon juice or vinegar.

New chains of franchised restaurants are spreading across the country that specialize in grilled chicken, with names like El Pollo Loco and Chicken on Fire. Order the breast of chicken, remove the skin and any excess fat, get a baked potato or an ear of corn, and you are home free. There is so much fat under the skin sometimes that it takes a half dozen or more napkins to remove the grease before you eat the chicken, but do it—it's worth the effort.

As mentioned in regard to Potato Day, many shopping malls have stands that sell baked potatoes. Get a plain po-tato and use your imitation butter sprinkle.

At your favorite pizza restaurant, order a vegetarian pizza with lots of fresh vegetables and lots of tomato sauce, and have them leave off the cheese. If prepared properly it is quite tasty.

11

START THE DAY RIGHT WITH BREAKFAST

A lot of people think that if they skip breakfast they are going to lose more weight. Wrong! Wrong! Wrong! Mother was right, it is best to start the day with a good breakfast. It is sort of like throwing a log on the fire to get the metabolism going in the morning. The embers have burned low during the night and in order to stoke the furnace and get the metabolism back in gear, you have to eat breakfast. It is important. Do it. *Eat breakfast.* On the Lifestyle or maintenance phase of this diet you have several choices for this meal. They are:

1. Oatmeal or other hot cereal
2. Shredded Wheat, Grape Nuts, Nutrigrain, Raisin Bran, or Health Valley Oat Bran Flakes; with skim/nonfat milk and fresh fruit
3. An egg-white omelette/frittata
4. Liquid protein drink, such as Slim-Fast made with skim milk, or Twinfast made with skim milk or water

5. Up to four pieces of fresh fruit

6. Six ounces of fresh juice and a muffin (see Christi's Basic Muffin Recipe, pages 122 and 266)

7. Six to eight ounces of nonfat yogurt, with a muffin or a piece of fruit

8. A cup of cooked brown rice with or without skim/nonfat milk and fruit

9. Any of the other breakfast suggestions from Jump-Start— e.g., vegetable soup, vegetables, corn on the cob, baked potato, etc.

12

WHAT TO
SNACK ON

It is okay to snack on the 1-Day-at-a-Time diet, as long as you follow these guidelines.

Snacks between Breakfast and Lunch

You don't have to snack. If you are not hungry, don't snack; if you are hungry, here is a list of healthy nutritious snacks:

BETWEEN BREAKFAST AND LUNCH (CHOOSE ONE)

1. Raw vegetables
2. Piece of fruit
3. Two low-salt or no-salt Chico San rice cakes
4. Glass of skim milk
5. Six to eight ounces of no-salt-added tomato or V8 juice
6. Two to four hard boiled egg whites

Snacks Between Lunch and Dinner

It is usually a good idea to have a snack late in the afternoon. It is a long time to go from lunch to dinner without stoking up the metabolism. Sometimes a piece of fruit, or raw vegetables, or rice cakes will do the trick. Sometimes a little heavier snack will take the edge off your afternoon hunger and keep you from being ravenous at dinnertime. So if you have had a lunch that has been mainly salad, you may find some cooked rice or a baked potato is a good late-afternoon snack. If you had heavier starches at lunch, you may only need to eat raw vegetables or a piece of fruit as your snack.

BETWEEN LUNCH AND DINNER (CHOOSE ONE)

1. Raw vegetables
2. Piece of fruit
3. Plain baked potato (with acceptable topping)
4. Two Chico San rice cakes
5. Cup of steamed rice
6. Unbuttered, unsalted *hot air*–popped corn
7. An ear of corn
8. Christi's bran muffin (see pages 122 and 266)
9. Two to four hard boiled egg whites

Please note that there are two bonus snack foods that are eaten only during Lifestyle—bran muffins and hot-air popcorn.

Snacks between Dinner and Bedtime

They say you lose more weight if you don't eat after dinnertime, and I am sure that is true, but I have never been able to do it. If I don't have a snack halfway between dinner and bedtime, I have trouble going to sleep. You have to be careful, though, because if you overdo the evening snack you can erase a lot of the good dieting work you have done during the day.

My favorite evening snack is hot-air popcorn. It is filling, delicious, and low in calories. If you don't add any butter or salt it is a healthy snack. You can try butter substitute sprinkles (Molly McButter, Butter Buds, Instead of Butter, and Best o' Butter), but these sprinkles won't stick to the popcorn so they give only a faint seasoning. You can have pretty much all you want of this hot-air popcorn.

If you cook vegetables for dinner, make extra. Steamed or stir-fried vegetables make an excellent snack between dinner and bedtime. They are quite filling and extremely low in calories. You can pretty much graze on them for a couple of hours and still lose weight.

BETWEEN DINNER AND BEDTIME (CHOOSE ONE)

1. Leftover cooked vegetables
2. Raw vegetables
3. Piece of fruit
4. Two or three Chico San rice cakes
5. Hot-air popcorn
6. Glass of skim milk
7. Glass of no-salt-added tomato or V8 juice
8. Five ounces of nonfat frozen yogurt
9. Two to four hard boiled egg whites

13

EXERCISE IS VITAL

At age 39 I had been smoking for 26 years and was unable to stop. Even a stint at Pritikin's as staff cardiologist was not enough to make me stop smoking. I made a deal with myself that by the time I reached the age of 40 I would be a nonsmoker. A few weeks before my birthday I was still smoking and I began to question my own integrity. Attending the annual meeting of the Association for Humanistic Psychology in San Diego, I noticed there was a seminar offered about running. I went out and bought a pair of running shoes, signed up for the program, stopped smoking, and began to exercise.

It was the most important moment of my life in terms of making positive choices for health. I had already handled the diet and nutrition part, but the exercise and smoking changes were transformational. I have never smoked since then. Unfortunately, I have had periods without exercise. And I have regretted every moment of those periods. From time to time I drift off the path and don't take the time or make the effort to exercise. And then when I begin to exercise again, I can't believe I let myself stray from the running path.

It doesn't make much difference what you do in terms of exercise. Like the Nike commercial says, just do it! However, there is a hierarchy of effective exercise. *Running* and *walking* are at the top of this hierarchy. Both are efficient ways to burn calories and to derive cardiovascular benefits. Running is more efficient than walking so you don't have to spend as much time running as you do walking, but they are equivalent in terms of their beneficial effects. One variation on the running theme is the *treadmill*. Another is the *trampoline* for rebounding and running in place. I am talking about the small type of trampoline that you can use in your living room in front of the television set and store under your couch or bed. *Bicycling* is another variation of the running/walking theme and can be done with a stationary bicycle or a free-wheeling bicycle. The new *stair-climbing machines*, such as Stair Master, are also excellent variations.

Tennis, squash, racquetball, handball, badminton, volleyball, and basketball are all acceptable forms of exercise. Swimming is terrific. Walking on the beach is wonderful. Dancing is divine.

You see, there is no excuse—there is something there for each and every one of us. We just have to get off our behinds and do it. Even if you want to stay on your behind, you can exercise on a bicycle.

How Much Exercise?

Some authorities say three times a week; others say four. My feeling is that exercise should be an integral part of every single day of your life. If you are out of shape, a smoker, or over 35, you should have a treadmill test before beginning an exercise program.

If you make exercise a part of your everyday routine you will find that your weight management will be easier. In fact, if you get only one thing from this book, I hope it's this: *Exercise, and eat according to the Master Plan (see page 151), and you will feel terrific and not only will you achieve a healthy weight, you will also minimize your risk of cardiovascular disease, cancer, diverticulitis, and a host of other maladies that fat flesh is heir to.*

How to Get Started on an Exercise Program

You can just start walking. Sounds very simple, doesn't it? Well, it is—just start walking. Start with a walk around the block and then gradually increase. Find a time that is convenient and do it every day. It is important and it will make you feel good.

Smoking and Exercise

Smoking and exercise do not go together well. When you smoke, carbon monoxide combines with your red blood cells and blocks their ability to release oxygen to the tissues. When you exercise you increase the oxygen demand of the tissues and increase the demand for the red blood cells to transfer oxygen. So when you begin to exercise, your smoking prevents your body from doing what it needs to do and you may harm yourself.

Just as tobacco smoke creates carbon monoxide that is poisonous to your body, exhaust fumes of cars will do the same thing. Whenever possible do your exercise away from exhaust fumes so you don't have to inhale carbon monoxide and put an added stress on your body.

NOW is a wonderful time to stop smoking, start exercising, and begin your diet all at the same time.

14

VITAMIN AND MINERAL SUPPLEMENTS

Nathan Pritikin believed that vitamin supplements are not necessary, that his diet provided all the vitamins and minerals needed. For many years I believed he was right and prescribed no vitamins and mineral supplements to my patients and did not use them myself. In recent years I have begun to prescribe vitamin and mineral supplements and have seen some rather dramatic results.

I do not believe in supernutrition and huge megadoses of vitamins and minerals, a la Durk Pearson and Sandy Shaw, but we do live in a polluted environment and there is now more than adequate evidence to support the beneficial use of certain vitamin and mineral supplements. Most important of these are the antioxidants. Antioxidants help our bodies fight pollutants. Primitive man, the basis of Pritikin's conceptualization, no longer exists. If there were no carbon monoxide, or polluted water, or pesticides in our food, as in the days of primitive man, we wouldn't need vitamin and mineral supplementation. But this is a dirty world we live in, highly stressful and highly polluted, and vitamin and mineral supplements can help our bodies deal with this environment.

Vitamin Supplementation

Vitamin A. There is really no need to supplement with vitamin A directly. If you ingest too much vitamin A it can be toxic. Small amounts of vitamin A are added to milk (skim/nonfat). The best way to obtain your requirement of vitamin A is from beta-carotene, which is the precursor of vitamin A. It is discussed below. If you do take a supplement with added vitamin A, there is no need to take more than 5,000 international units (IUs) per day.

Vitamin D. I do not recommend that you take any vitamin D supplementation. Ten minutes a day in the sun activates your body's own natural vitamin D. Just like vitamin A, vitamin D is added to milk. If you drink as much as four glasses of milk (skim/nonfat) a day you will have all the vitamin D you need. If you take excessive vitamin D you run the risk of facilitating calcification in places in your body where you don't want calcification—such as inside your arteries.

Vitamin E. Vitamin E is an important supplement that has antioxidant properties. Vitamin E is a fat-soluble vitamin, and since we are going to be limiting the fats on this diet, it is beneficial to take vitamin E as a supplement. I recommend that you supplement your diet with 200–300 IUs of vitamin E per day.

Vitamin C. Without any doubt we should all supplement our diet with vitamin C. Vitamin C is a powerful antioxidant and may be one of the most useful antioxidants because it plays a multiplicity of roles in the body. It can't be stored by the body so it must be taken every day, preferably in two to three divided doses throughout the day. I find if I take vitamin C after dinner it has a stimulatory effect and will sometimes cause insomnia, so I suggest that you not take vitamin C supplements near bedtime. One gram (1,000 milligrams) of vitamin C daily is my recommended supplementation.

Vitamin B₁ (Thiamine). Thiamine is an important vitamin necessary for carbohydrate metabolism, and you should supplement your high-complex-carbohydrate diet with it. My recommendation is up to 50 milligrams of thiamine per day.

Vitamin B₂ (Riboflavin). Riboflavin is also a useful vitamin to supplement and is a co-factor for some of the antioxidants. Vitamin B₂ is what causes the urine to turn yellow-orange when it is excreted by the kidneys. One of my nutritionist friends says that he knows his patients are taking enough riboflavin when they report that their urine shows the yellow-orange color through a good bit of the day. I recommend that you take up to 50 milligrams of riboflavin each day.

Vitamin B₃ (Niacin-Nicotinamide). Niacin or vitamin B₃ is an important vitamin and has been used therapeutically to lower serum cholesterol and triglyceride levels. The problem with supplementing niacin is that it cannot be taken on an empty stomach or in too large a dose or it will cause extreme flushing and itching of the skin. I recommend niacin supplementation at the level of 100 milligrams a day. If you have high blood cholesterol or high triglycerides, consult your physician about the possibility of using niacin to help lower cholesterol and triglycerides. In all likelihood the 1-Day-at-a-Time diet will have a pronounced beneficial effect on lowering your cholesterol and triglycerides, and only a few dozen people in a thousand will need further niacin supplementation for this purpose.

One of my patients recently reported that before beginning the 1-Day-at-a-Time diet he had been prescribed medication to reduce his cholesterol level of over 300 mg/dl, a dangerously high level. After following the 1-Day-at-a-Time diet for only three weeks, his cholesterol fell to 130 mg/dl. His physician discontinued the medication. One month later, on no medication and following the Lifestyle phase of the diet, his cholesterol was 180.

This is an example of hundreds of cases of dangerously high cholesterol values being converted to extremely healthy ones by diet alone.

If you are currently on medication for elevated cholesterol, *do not stop this medication on your own*. Consult your physician for a repeat blood test after you have been on the diet for three or four weeks.

Pantothenic Acid. Pantothenic acid, which used to be called vitamin B_5, is a useful supplement. It may be beneficial in adaptation to stress. I recommend supplementation at the 200–250 milligrams level.

Vitamin B_6 (Pyridoxine). Vitamin B_6 is a cofactor in many important chemical reactions in the body and is a useful vitamin to supplement. There is proven toxicity with excessive amounts of vitamin B_6 (2,000–6,000 milligrams per day). I recommend supplementation of vitamin B_6 not to exceed 50 milligrams a day.

Beta-Carotene. Beta-carotene is the precursor of vitamin A. Whereas vitamin A in excessive amounts may be toxic, beta-carotene has had no proven toxicity. The body simply stops converting beta-carotene to vitamin A when enough has been ingested. Beta-carotene has been shown to be an important antioxidant and it is believed to be a cancer preventive. There is a study going on that will answer the question whether beta-carotene does in fact prevent cancer. I recommend supplementation with beta-carotene at the level of 25,000 international units per day.

Other Supplements. There are numerous other supplements and vitamins that may be beneficial, but the evidence is not clear. If you choose to supplement these nutrients the safe values are:

- Folic acid—400 micrograms per day
- Vitamin B$_{12}$—50–100 micrograms per day
- Bioflavonoids—200–600 milligrams per day
- Fish oil (maxEPA)—300–1,000 milligrams per day

Mineral Supplementation

Calcium. Calcium is an important supplement. Without sufficient calcium in the diet, our bones will become brittle and break. Recent data also suggest that calcium may help prevent colon cancer. If you drink four glasses of skim milk a day you will get all the calcium you need and will not need to supplement. Yogurt is also rich in calcium and the calcium is more concentrated in yogurt than in milk. If you use nonfat yogurt or nonfat frozen yogurt in your diet, your need to supplement with calcium will be diminished by the amount of calcium you take in. Total intake of calcium should add up to at least 1,000 milligrams a day.

Magnesium. Magnesium is needed as a balance to calcium. If you take calcium supplements, use one that also contains magnesium.

Selenium. Selenium is an important mineral that has strong antioxidant properties. It is difficult to recommend precise selenium supplementation because some areas of the country have soil that is rich in selenium and some areas are selenium poor. Too much selenium may be toxic. Fifty to 100 micrograms per day is my recommendation.

Zinc. Zinc is an important cofactor for many important chemical reactions in the body. This mineral must be supplemented with caution. Excessive amounts of zinc may lower levels of "good" cholesterol (HDL). My recommendation is that zinc supplementation not exceed the recommended daily allowance of 15 milligrams per day.

Chromium. Chromium is an essential mineral that is very beneficial in some people in helping to stabilize carbohydrate metabolism. I recommend supplementation with 200 milligrams per day.

Other Minerals. I do not recommend supplementation with copper, iron, manganese, or molybdenum, unless you have documented deficiencies of these minerals.

Vitamin Allergies. Many vitamins are made from yeast, and many people have a low-grade allergy to yeast. I recommend that you use a yeast-free vitamin supplement to minimize your risk of yeast allergy. The label should say "yeast-free."

What Do I Take?

There are so many vitamins available on the market that it is difficult for me to tell you exactly which ones to take. Perhaps just telling you what I take will give you the reference you need to make your own choice.

I take one capsule of Twin Lab MaxiLife Capsules a day. This vitamin has the whole spectrum of vitamins and antioxidants. The manufacturer recommends taking four per day, but I get some other antioxidants from another source, which I will tell you about in a moment. Be sure not to take the MaxiLife on an empty stomach, because as the manufacturer states in red on the label, the niacin (vitamin B$_3$) may cause a flush. So when you take the MaxiLife or other vitamins with niacin in them, be sure to take them with food. You could use only MaxiLife, taking four capsules a day as the manufacturer recommends, and satisfy your total vitamin supplementation. Many of you will elect to do this for convenience.

I complement my MaxiLife by taking two Anti-Ox capsules each day. Anti-Ox is a formulation by the Allergy Research Group in San Leandro, California, that contains all of the essential antioxidants. It has two less important antioxidants that MaxiLife doesn't have, but it doesn't have all of the B vitamins and minerals that MaxiLife does have.

I also take one Country Life chelated calcium-magnesium-potassium tablet per day. This provides 500 milligrams of calcium. I get my additional calcium and magnesium from skim milk and nonfat yogurt. I take two capsules of Twin Lab's C Plus Citrus Bioflavonoids. This provides bioflavonoids and 1,000 milligrams of vitamin C per day.

Basic Vitamin Supplements

If you find these instructions for figuring out your vitamin supplementation too difficult, just take one of the basic supplements, such as One-a-Day vitamins, Centrum, or Theragran.

15

USE YOUR MIND TO HELP HEAL YOUR BODY

When we come into this world we are all skinny, innocent, and needy of love. As we grow older and larger, we lose some of the innocence and we don't always find all the love we need in our life. We reach out for love, positive regard, and "strokes," and sometimes they just aren't there. So we turn to the most available source of nourishment: it is often behind the refrigerator or pantry door. Food is stimulating, easily available, and at some superficial level of our being it is satisfying, at least for the time being. So we substitute food for the love and psychological nourishment that is not so readily available. Because some of the desire pangs in our stomach are eased, we return to this source over and over again when what we really need is to be loved.

Love Yourself More

So the vicious cycle continues; seeking more nourishment and love from food—getting fatter, getting more unhappy, disapproving of oneself. In order to free yourself from this cycle, you must learn to love yourself and to recognize that fatty, creamy, rich, luscious food doesn't have anything to do with what you really need and want—nutritionally or spiritually. The first step in any diet is the acknowledgment of self—that "I am worthy," that "I deserve love," that "I am lovable," and "I care about me." That which we love we will do anything for; we will make any sacrifice for those we love. So in loving ourselves we commit to ourselves and acknowledge that we are willing to make sacrifices necessary to be successful on this diet. Just as we each have our own biochemical individuality, and some of us can eat fruit and others can't, some can eat dairy products and others can't, we have our own spiritual individuality as well.

One of my favorite quotes is by John Lilly, M.D.: "That which we believe to be true, either is true or becomes true in our own mind." So you see, with just a slight shift of consciousness your belief system can become one of a loving, radiant, healthy, lean, lovable, joyous being. It takes absolutely no more energy to hold this belief system than destructive, self-limiting beliefs. Sometimes when we start loving ourselves we find that the environment we have been living in is not a loving one. It may be too noisy, too polluted, or our boss may be too critical or negative. Sometimes with this very slight shift of consciousness, this new belief system, this affirmative action so to speak, we find that in loving ourselves we make changes in our life that actually support that loving. Not only a change in eating habits to a more nourishing, or a kinder, gentler diet; we can also try to make our world a kinder, gentler world, one that supports and nourishes us just as the diet does. You will only be overweight as long as you believe that you must be overweight. Use these tools that I have provided you with in this book as stepping stones to a new, happier, and leaner you.

The Master Plan

Putting It All Together

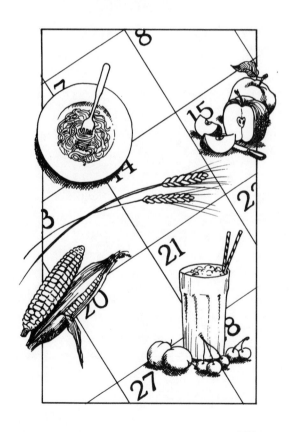

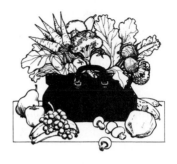

If you have been reading this book and have stayed with me until now, you already know much of what is coming up. This is a plan that you can live with, and it's a plan that can help you to live. The Master Plan outlined here summarizes how to do this program.

Exercise

In order to achieve optimum health and to maximize your opportunity to lose weight on this diet, *you need to exercise.* It doesn't have to be complicated. Just start walking. If you are not in shape at all and you haven't been on an exercise program, walk at a slow pace for a few minutes each day. It doesn't have to be much—just start doing it. Five minutes. Ten minutes. Fifteen or 20 minutes, or if you are in better shape, start with a 30-minute walk. Make it slow and easy. Don't wear yourself out and don't try to work up a sweat when you first start. Just start a walking program and do what you can, even if it means walking halfway around the block and turning around and coming back. Just get started on your walk and then each day go a little farther, do a little bit more. If you start with 5 minutes a day the first week, increase it to 10 minutes the second week. If you start with 15 minutes a day the first week, go to 20 minutes the next week. As you begin to lose weight your energy will increase and you will be able to do more with less effort.

If you have a history of cardiovascular disease or high blood pressure, or if you are over 35, check with your doctor before you start the exercise program.

For those of you who are younger and healthier and in better shape, you can start a little bit more vigorous exercise program customized to your current level of fitness. If you are over 35 and you want to start a vigorous exercise program, see your doctor first and get an exercise test during cardiac monitoring. This is good insurance against having a heart attack on your exercise program.

If you are a smoker, *stop smoking*, then begin your exercise program. In fact, the exercise program and the diet together will help you stop smoking. *Reread "How to Use This Diet"* (see page 15).

Vitamins

I want you to take vitamins on this program, especially the antioxidant vitamins, because I believe they will help you feel better and will protect you and help you live a longer, healthier life. You can customize the vitamin program with the individual components I have listed in the section on vitamin and mineral supplements (see page 142), or you can take a good multivitamin supplement containing between 10 and 50 milligrams of the B vitamins per day. Vitamins E and C are important too. You may want to consult a professional nutritionist to help you customize your vitamin program.

How Much Animal Protein Do You Really Need?

Some people need more protein than others. I have seen people eating excessive amounts of animal protein and I have recommended that they become vegetarians and eat no animal protein for a period of time; this has proven to be a very useful and healthy therapeutic strategy for them. By the same token, I have seen vegetarians who were failing to thrive and I have recommended that they add animal protein to their diet. Often they made this addition very reluctantly because of preconceived ideas, only to find that the addition of animal protein is energizing and revitalizing to their system. We cannot decide on an intellectual level what we will eat. Our biochemical individuality and uniqueness will determine what is best for us to eat, and this will vary at different times in our lives.

You must pay attention to your body and use your intuition, be flexible, and be willing to change. There was a point in my life when I decided that I must become a vegetarian and eat no animal protein in order to reduce my serum cholesterol and clean my arteries. During this phase, my nails became so soft that they peeled off, my vital energy became very low, and a running injury would not heal. I was protein-deficient, but I didn't listen to my body. It has taken me a long time to learn that, and I've tried to share some of what I have learned with you. So some of you will need to eat a full eight ounces of animal protein each day. I believe that better than 99 percent of you will have adequate protein intake with eight ounces of animal protein a day or less. Many of you will get all the protein you need by eating chicken or fish only a couple of times a week; others will do just fine with animal protein three or four times a week. As you can see, it is impossible for me to make one prescription that applies to every single person. Be flexible, listen to your body, and use moderation.

Remember, one of the main reasons to limit the amount of animal protein in your diet is that cholesterol is found only in animal flesh. Even if you eat the more healthy fish and fowl, it still contains cholesterol. Egg whites, skim milk, and nonfat yogurt are free of cholesterol, however.

What Amount of Carbohydrates Can You Eat and Still Lose Weight?

I want you to use the carbohydrate choices, that is, rice, corn, beans, peas, potatoes, and pasta in the Lifestyle section—as a reward for your exercise. If you don't exercise and eat the carbohydrates, it will be difficult for you to lose weight. So why not try limiting yourself to one carbohydrate serving for each 30 minutes of exercise you engage in each day? If you don't exercise regularly, eat more vegetables and omit the carbohydrates; you will lose more weight on the 1-Day-at-a-Time diet if you do this.

Lifestyle Master Plan Menu

Again, reread Chapter 2, "How to Use This Diet" (see page 15). The Lifestyle phase menu plan that follows is the menu plan that you'll stay with for the rest of your life, in order to continue to lose weight and to consolidate your weight loss. If you wish, you can begin this diet with Lifestyle, as I mentioned earlier. Your weight loss will not be quite as rapid as it would be if you used Jump-Start, but it will be acceptable and very beneficial.

BREAKFAST (CHOOSE ONE)

1. Oatmeal or other hot cereal
2. Shredded Wheat, Grape Nuts, Nutri-grain, Raisin Bran, or Health Valley Oat Bran Flakes; with skim/nonfat milk and fresh fruit
3. An egg-white omelette/frittata or hard-boiled egg whites
4. Liquid protein drink such as Slim-Fast, made with skim milk or Twinfast, made with nonfat milk or water.

5. Up to four pieces of fresh fruit
6. Six ounces of fresh juice and a muffin (see Christi's Basic Muffin Recipe, pages 122 and 266)
7. Six to eight ounces of nonfat yogurt, with a muffin or a piece of fruit
8. A cup of cooked brown rice with or without skim/nonfat milk and fruit
9. A baked potato, an ear or two of corn, or cooked vegetables
10. A bowl of soup or a bowl of pasta

SNACK BETWEEN BREAKFAST AND LUNCH (CHOOSE ONE)

1. Raw vegetables
2. Piece of fruit
3. Two low-salt or no-salt *Chico San* rice cakes
4. Glass of skim milk
5. Six to eight ounces of no-salt-added tomato or V8 juice
6. Two to four hard boiled egg whites

LUNCH OR DINNER

1. Large salad with reduced calorie/no-oil salad dressing (may add two chopped hard-boiled egg whites)
2. Protein (maximum of eight ounces per day)
   a. Fish
   b. Defatted and skinned turkey or chicken breast
   c. Egg-white omelette
3. Cooked vegetables
4. Soup
5. Carbohydrate (choose one):
   a. Corn
   b. Pasta
   c. Rice
   d. Potato
   e. Beans, peas, legumes

(The choices for lunch and dinner are identical. Some people prefer to eat a heavier lunch and lighter dinner, while others do it vice versa. You will always want to have a large salad, either as your whole meal or as an appetizer, at lunch and dinner. If you have the salad as your entire meal, you may add protein either in the form of diced chicken or turkey breast, skinned and defatted; or hard-boiled egg whites; or fish, such as water-packed white albacore tuna that has been drained. If you use the salad as an appetizer without the added protein, you may have a protein entrée of either broiled, baked, or otherwise cooked fish, or defatted, skinned chicken or turkey breast, and then have a side dish of cooked vegetables and a starch. Another alternative would be a salad, soup, and a baked potato. Steamed or stir-fried vegetables and brown rice is another option. As you can see, we are getting back to the same ideas suggested for Mix and Match Day.)

SNACK BETWEEN LUNCH AND DINNER (CHOOSE ONE)

1. Raw vegetables
2. Piece of fruit
3. Plain baked potato (with acceptable topping)
4. Two Chico San rice cakes
5. Cup of steamed rice
6. Unbuttered, unsalted *hot-air*–popped corn
7. An ear of corn
8. Christi's bran muffin (see pages 122 and 266)
9. Two to four hard boiled egg whites

NOTE: There are two bonus snack foods that are eaten only during Lifestyle—bran muffins and hot-air popcorn.

SNACK BETWEEN DINNER AND BEDTIME (CHOOSE ONE)

1. Leftover cooked vegetables
2. Raw vegetables

3. Piece of fruit
4. Two or three Chico San rice cakes
5. Hot-air popcorn
6. Glass of skim milk
7. Glass of no-salt-added tomato or V8 juice
8. Five ounces of nonfat frozen yogurt
9. Two to four hard boiled egg whites

Recipes

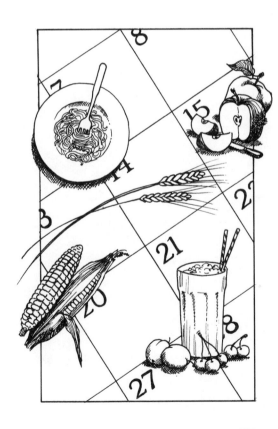

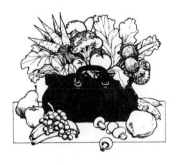

The recipes in this section were all created by my mother, Edythe. When I joined the staff of Nathan Pritikin at his Longevity Center in Santa Barbara in 1977 and began to see some of the magical things that diet and nutrition could accomplish, I realized that it could be a life-saving experience for my mother. At that time she was quite ill, suffering from angina pectoris and the effects of a mild heart attack, as well as chronic pancreatitis. When I saw the dramatic improvements that people with similar problems were experiencing at the Pritikin Center, I told Nathan Pritikin about my mother's predicament and he invited her to come to the Center as his guest. She spent 28 days in the program, and as a result of that experience was able to turn her health around dramatically.

Being the good Jewish mother that she is, Edythe went home and began working on recipes of her own in order to make healthful eating more delicious and exciting. The recipes that follow in this section are a gift from my mother to you.

These recipes can all be used in the Lifestyle phase of the 1-Day-at-a-Time diet. Some have been used during the one-food-a-day Jump-Start phase. These are easily identified by an asterisk next to the name of the recipe. All of the recipes follow the principles of healthy eating; that is, they adhere to the principles of low fat, high complex carbohydrates, unprocessed natural foods, free of sugar and refined products, and high in fiber.

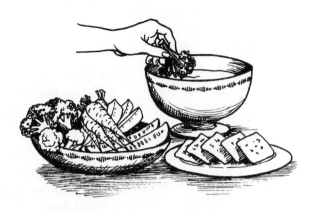

Appetizers

Garbanzo (Chick-pea) Dip

2 cups cooked garbanzo beans, drained (save liquid)
½ cup plain nonfat yogurt
¼ cup chopped parsley
¼ cup sliced green onions
2 cloves garlic, peeled and crushed
Juice of 1 lemon
⅛ teaspoon ground cumin
Dash of white pepper

Combine all ingredients in the bowl of the food processor. Using the metal blade, process with on-and-off turns until completely mixed and smooth. If too thick add reserved liquid, a teaspoon at a time. Serve with cucumber sticks, celery sticks, carrot sticks, and cherry tomatoes or rice cakes. Yields about 2 cups.

Yogurt Dip

1 cup plain nonfat yogurt
½ cup dry-curd or low-fat cottage cheese, mashed
2 tablespoons finely chopped cucumber
1 clove garlic, mashed

Mix all ingredients together and refrigerate at least 2 hours. Good to serve as an hors d'oeuvre dip. Yields about 1½ cups. The dip can be thinned with nonfat milk and used as a salad dressing.

Mexican Bean Dip

2 cups cooked garbanzo beans, drained
2 cups cooked pinto beans
1½ cups chopped fresh tomatoes
¼ cup sliced green pepper
¼ cup sliced green onions
2 tablespoons Ortega green chili peppers
1½ teaspoons fresh lemon juice
1 tablespoon ground cumin
Dash of Tabasco sauce

Combine all ingredients in a blender or food processor. Process until desired consistency is reached. Adjust seasonings to taste. Serve with assorted raw vegetables. Yields 4 cups.

Cheese Spread

2 cups dry-curd or drained low-fat cottage cheese or hoop cheese

2 teaspoons skim milk

2 teaspoons dried minced onion

2 teaspoons fresh lemon juice

Place ingredients in blender or processor and blend until smooth, about 1 minute. Adjust to desired consistency by adding milk, a little at a time. Serve as a dip with raw vegetables. Yields 2 cups.

Eggplant Spread

1 medium eggplant

1 medium onion, finely chopped

1 clove garlic, mashed

1 tablespoon lemon juice

Red onion rings

Cherry tomatoes

Bake eggplant for 40–45 minutes in a 350°F. oven. When it is tender to the touch, remove from oven and allow to cool for 5 minutes. Peel off the skin with a wet knife. Place eggplant in a bowl and mash, or use food processor. Add onion, garlic, and lemon juice. Mix well and chill. Garnish with red onion rings and cherry tomatoes. Yields ½ cup.

Cream Cheese Substitute

Place 8 oz. dry-curd or low-fat cottage cheese in a blender or food processor. Add nonfat milk 1 tablespoon at a time and blend until desired consistency. If desired, add:

1 tablespoon grated cucumber
1 clove garlic, minced
½ teaspoon fresh lemon juice
½ teaspoon dillweed

Refrigerate for several hours to allow flavors to marry. To use as a dressing, add more skim milk and blend thoroughly. Yields approx. 2 cups.

Yogurt Cream Cheese

Place 1 cup plain nonfat yogurt in several thicknesses of cheesecloth and place over a bowl. Secure the cheesecloth with a rubber band. Allow to drain completely. Store in the refrigerator overnight. Remove yogurt from cheesecloth and mix well with seasoning of your choice: dash of onion powder and dash of garlic powder; a sprinkle of dillweed; or nutmeg, cinnamon, or ginger. Yields 1 cup.

Dill and Curry Cheese Spread

1 cup dry-curd or low-fat cottage cheese
2 tablespoons plain nonfat yogurt
1 tablespoon finely chopped fresh dillweed
½ teaspoon curry powder
¼ teaspoon dry mustard
   Nonfat milk (optional)

Mash cottage cheese with yogurt and place in blender. Add dill, curry powder, and mustard. Blend thoroughly. If necessary, add a little nonfat milk for spreading consistency. Yields approx. 1 cup.

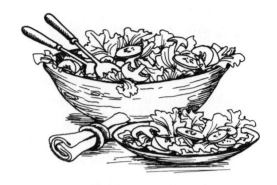

Salads

Helpful Hints for Salad Making

Select fresh salad greens. For interesting contrast, use different varieties—don't overlook watercress, chicory, and endive.

Never soak salad greens. Wash them carefully so as not to break the veins; rinse and trim under cold running water. To drain excess water from greens, either pat dry with a clean kitchen towel or paper towel, or whirl dry in a salad spinner. Arrange greens loosely in a refrigerator pan so excess water drains from them while they are crisping. Chill salad ingredients a few hours before serving.

Break or tear greens into bite-sized pieces. Cut head lettuce in quarters, then break apart. Toss salad or combine ingredients and dressing just before serving. Salad plates should be chilled at least three hours prior to the meal; salad dressing should be chilled at least two hours.

Colorful garnishes make salads more appetizing. Try using the whites of hard-boiled eggs, tomato wedges, sliced radishes, sliced green pepper, raw asparagus, carrots, or cauliflower. Red or pink beans or garbanzo beans may be spooned over the salad for a festive and tasty finishing touch.

Garbanzo and Kidney Bean Salad

1½ cups cooked garbanzos, drained
1½ cups cooked red kidney beans, drained
 1 cup diced celery
 ½ cup diced green pepper
 ¼ cup pimiento
 ⅛ teaspoon white pepper
 1 cup plain nonfat yogurt
 2 tablespoons horseradish

Combine all ingredients except yogurt and horseradish. Mix the yogurt and horseradish together. Add to the bean mixture. Chill. Serve on crisp lettuce leaves. Yields 6–8 servings.

Kidney Bean and Tuna Salad

 1 6½-oz. can water-packed tuna, drained
 2 cups cooked kidney beans, drained and chilled
 ½ cup finely sliced celery
 ½ cup chopped green onions
 ¼ cup finely chopped green pepper
   No-oil Italian dressing
   Hard-boiled egg whites, quartered

Combine all ingredients except dressing. Add dressing and toss lightly. Garnish with quartered hard-boiled egg whites (discard yolks). Serve on crisp lettuce. Yields 4 servings.

Spaghetti Squash Salad*

½ cup cooked spaghetti squash[1]
1 cup diced cooked chicken breast, skinned, all visible fat removed
½ cup thinly sliced celery
½ cup plain nonfat yogurt
Juice of 1 lemon
1 tablespoon pimiento
1 teaspoon vinegar
¼ teaspoon Italian herb seasoning
Cherry tomatoes
Green pepper strips

Combine all ingredients except tomatoes and green pepper; toss lightly with two forks. Adjust seasoning to taste. Chill before serving. Garnish with halved cherry tomatoes and green pepper strips. Serve over a bed of greens. Yields 4–6 servings.

[1] See basic cooking instructions, page 245.

Tossed Salad with Tuna*

1 6½-oz. can water-packed solid white albacore tuna, drained
4 cups mixed salad greens
1 cup sliced green onions
1 green pepper, cut in sticks
½ cup sliced radishes
1 cucumber, cut in sticks
2 carrots, cut in sticks
Cherry tomatoes or tomato wedges

Combine all ingredients except tomatoes in a large bowl; toss. Garnish with cherry tomatoes or tomato wedges. Serve with lemon juice, vinegar, or your favorite no-oil dressing. Yields 4 servings.

Beet Salad

1¼ cups diced cooked beets
4 teaspoons chopped onions
4 teaspoons plain nonfat yogurt
⅛ teaspoon ground cloves
Dash of allspice

Combine all ingredients. Chill and serve on salad greens. Yields 4 servings.

Vegetable and Brown Rice Salad*

1 cup fresh chop suey vegetables
⅓ cup sliced mushrooms
2 green onions, sliced
1 teaspoon no-oil Italian dressing
½ teaspoon Tamari sauce
⅛ teaspoon dry mustard
⅛ teaspoon ground ginger
1 cup cooked brown rice

Combine all ingredients except rice. Chill and serve over the rice. Yields 2 servings.

Cucumber Delight

1 medium cucumber, sliced
1 teaspoon plain nonfat yogurt
1 teaspoon sliced green onions
1 teaspoon tomato paste
⅛ teaspoon ground cumin
Dash of white pepper

Combine all ingredients. Chill. Serve on crisp lettuce leaves. Yields 2 servings.

Cottage Cheese Garden Salad

½ cup dry-curd or nonfat cottage cheese
2 tablespoons plain nonfat yogurt
2 tablespoons chopped green onions
2 tablespoons chopped green pepper
2 tablespoons chopped radishes
1 rib celery, chopped
⅛ teaspoon garlic powder
Dash of white pepper

Combine cottage cheese and yogurt; mix well. Combine remaining ingredients; add to cheese mixture. Toss lightly. Serve on crisp salad greens. Yields 2 servings.

Radish and Cucumber Salad

½ cup plain nonfat yogurt
1 tablespoon apple cider vinegar
1 tablespoon pimiento

2 cups cucumbers, halved lengthwise and seeded
½ cup sliced radishes
Parsley or mint sprigs

Combine yogurt, vinegar, and pimiento in blender. Blend until smooth. Pour over cucumbers and radishes. Toss lightly. Chill. Garnish with sprigs of mint or parsley. Yields 4 servings.

Green Salad Mold

1 envelope unflavored gelatin
⅛ teaspoon white pepper
1¾ cups water, divided
¼ cup apple cider vinegar
1 tablespoon lemon juice
1 cup shredded raw spinach
1 cup chopped celery
¼ cup grated carrots
¼ cup chopped green onions
Cherry tomatoes, halved
Cucumber slices

Mix gelatin with white pepper in saucepan. Add ½ cup water. Place over low heat and stir constantly until gelatin is dissolved. Remove from heat. Stir in the remaining 1¼ cups of water, vinegar, and lemon juice. Chill to consistency of unbeaten egg whites. Fold in spinach, celery, carrots, and green onions. Pour into a 4-cup mold or individual molds. Chill until firm. To unmold, follow instructions from Waldorf Salad (next recipe). Garnish with cherry tomato halves and crinkle-sliced cucumbers. Yields 6 servings.

Confetti Coleslaw

1 small head cabbage
2 medium carrots, peeled
6 radishes (remove tops)
1 green pepper (remove seeds)
1 small cucumber
½ cup scallions
2 small Jalapeño peppers, chopped (optional)
  yogurt cream cheese (page 168) diluted with skim milk

Quarter and core cabbage. Chop cabbage, carrots, radishes, green pepper, cucumber, and scallions (white and green ends) into small pieces. In a large bowl, combine all ingredients and toss thoroughly. Add enough yogurt cream cheese to obtain desired consistency. Yields 10–12 servings.

Waldorf Salad

1 envelope unflavored gelatin
1½ cups water, divided
¼ cup fresh lemon juice
2 cups chopped Red or Golden Delicious apples
½ cup diced celery
¼ cup water chestnuts, drained and chopped
1 banana
  Other fruit for garnish (optional)

In a saucepan, add ½ cup water to the gelatin. Place over low heat and stir constantly until gelatin is completely dissolved. Remove from heat. Stir in the remaining cup of water and the lemon juice. Chill mixture to consistency of unbeaten egg whites. Fold in apples, celery, and water chestnuts. Rinse a 4-cup mold with cold water; do not dry. Pour salad mixture into mold and refrigerate until firm.

To unmold, dip mold in warm water. Loosen gelatin around the edge with tip of a paring knife. Place a serving dish on top of the mold and turn upside down. Shake while holding dish tightly to the mold.

For a garnish, run the prongs of a fork lengthwise down a peeled banana, then slice the banana crosswise to form crinkly-edged rounds. Add any other fruit you desire. Yields 6 servings.

Corn Salad

    1 medium green pepper
    3 cups cooked corn kernels
 1½ cups thinly sliced celery
    3 green onions, chopped
    2 tablespoons chopped sweet pickle
  ⅔ cup plain nonfat yogurt
    1 tablespoon vinegar
  ½ teaspoon unsalted prepared mustard
  ¼ teaspoon crushed basil leaves
  ⅛ teaspoon white pepper
      Pimiento strips

Cut green pepper in half and remove seeds. Chop one-half the pepper; reserve other half. In a bowl, combine corn, celery, chopped green pepper, onions, and pickle. Cover and chill. In a small bowl, combine the yogurt, vinegar, mustard, basil, and white pepper. Cover and chill. Before serving, combine all ingredients except the other half of the green pepper. Arrange salad on lettuce leaves. Slice pepper into strips. Garnish salad with green pepper strips and pimiento strips. Yields 6 servings.

Cottage Cheese and Beet Salad

1 envelope unflavored gelatin
1½ cups water, divided
¼ cup fresh lemon juice
1 cup chopped cooked beets
1 cup dry-curd cottage cheese
Salad greens

In a saucepan, add ½ cup water to the gelatin. Place over low heat and stir constantly until gelatin is dissolved. Remove from heat. Stir in remaining 1 cup of water and the lemon juice. Chill to consistency of unbeaten egg whites. Fold in beets and cottage cheese. Pour into a 3-cup mold and chill until firm. Unmold on serving dish and garnish with salad greens. Yields 4 servings.

Perfection Salad

1 envelope gelatin
1 cup water, divided
1 6-oz. can apple juice concentrate, thawed
¼ cup vinegar
1 tablespoon fresh lemon juice
¾ cup finely shredded cabbage
1 cup diced celery
1 pimiento, chopped

In a saucepan, sprinkle gelatin in ½ cup water to soften. Over low heat, stir until gelatin is dissolved. Remove from heat. Add remaining water, apple juice concentrate, vinegar, and lemon juice. Chill to consistency of unbeaten egg whites. Fold in cabbage, celery, and pimiento. Pour into 3-cup mold or individual molds. Chill until firm. Yields 6 servings.

Vegetable Salad with Curry Dressing

2 cups each, raw or cooked vegetables, cut up into bite-size pieces and combined in a salad bowl (cabbage, tomatoes, cucumbers, and zucchini, or any other vegetables you prefer)

DRESSING

1 cup plain nonfat yogurt

1 tablespoon curry powder

1 tablespoon apple cider vinegar

1 clove garlic, mashed

Combine ingredients and pour over the vegetables. Toss gently and serve. Yields 4 servings.

Curried Chicken and Sweet Potato Salad

3 lbs. sweet potatoes, washed well

3 cups cubed cooked chicken breast, skinned, all visible fat removed

1 20-oz. can unsweetened pineapple chunks, completely drained

1 large green pepper, cut into thin strips

½ cup sliced green onions

½ cup currants

In a large saucepan, boil enough water to cover the sweet potatoes. Carefully drop the potatoes into the water and return to a boil. Cover, reduce heat, and simmer for 25–30 minutes until potatoes are barely tender. *Do not overcook.* Cool, peel, halve, and slice ¼ inch thick. Combine with the chicken, drained pineapple, green pepper, green onions, and currants. Toss with Curry Dressing (see recipe below). Cover and refrigerate several hours or overnight, allowing the flavors to marry. Yields 6–8 servings.

Curry Dressing

⅓ cup apple juice concentrate, thawed
⅓ cup white wine vinegar
1 tablespoon soy sauce or Tamari sauce
2 tablespoons curry powder
1 clove garlic, crushed
¼ teaspoon ground cumin
¼ teaspoon onion powder
Dash of picante sauce

Combine all ingredients in a jar with a tight-fitting lid. Shake well and chill.

Green Bean Salad

1 lb. green beans
2 heads romaine lettuce, cut into pieces
1 lb. carrots, shredded
1 lb. snow peas
2 pints cherry tomatoes
4 medium-size onions, thinly sliced

Wash and cut ends off of the green beans. Parboil 4–6 minutes. Drain and plunge into ice water to set color. Combine remaining ingredients and chill thoroughly. Pour dressing (see recipe below) over green beans and toss lightly. Yields 6 servings.

Vinaigrette Dressing

4 tablespoons vinegar of your choice
2 tablespoons finely chopped parsley
1 tablespoon apple juice concentrate, thawed

With a wire whisk, mix ingredients. Yields 1 cup.

Garbanzo and Bulgur Wheat Salad

½ cup uncooked bulgur wheat
1 cup boiling water
½ cup fresh lemon juice
¼ cup no-oil Italian dressing
1 cup cooked garbanzos, drained
1 cup sliced mushrooms
½ cup finely chopped parsley
½ cup sliced carrots
½ cup sliced green onions
Cucumber slices and tomato wedges

Place bulgur wheat in a large heatproof bowl. Pour boiling water over the bulgur wheat; toss to moisten evenly. Cover bowl and allow the bulgur wheat to expand for 1 hour. Pour lemon juice and dressing over the bulgur; mix with a fork. Layer each vegetable on top of the bulgur mixture. Cover and refrigerate for several hours. Toss before serving. Garnish with cucumber slices and tomato wedges. Yields 8 servings.

Stuffed Tomatoes*

2 medium tomatoes

½ cup diced cooked chicken breast, skinned, all visible fat removed

1 tablespoon chopped green onion

1 rib celery, chopped

1 teaspoon chopped green pepper

3 teaspoons no-oil Italian dressing

1 teaspoon picante sauce (mild)

⅛ teaspoon white pepper

Dash of ground thyme

Hollow out the tomatoes. Chop the flesh and reserve the hollowed-out shells. Lightly toss together chopped tomatoes and all other ingredients. Fill tomato shells with the mixture. Serve on crisp lettuce leaves. Yields 2 servings.

Stuffed Papaya with Chicken

1½ lbs. boneless breast of chicken, shredded, skinned all visible fat removed

¼ cup chicken stock

¾ cup thinly sliced green pepper

¼ cup chopped onion

¼ cup very finely chopped gingerroot, or 1 scant teaspoon ground ginger

⅓ cup dry sherry

6 tablespoons Tomato Ketchup (see page 226)

1 tablespoon thinly sliced red chili pepper (optional)

3 medium-size very ripe papayas, cut in half

Sauté shredded chicken in 3 tablespoons chicken stock. In a separate nonstick skillet, sauté the green pepper, onions, and ginger in the remaining chicken stock until the peppers begin to soften. Add sherry, ketchup, and sautéed chicken. Simmer for 2 minutes. Add red chili and stir lightly. Preheat oven to 350°F. Bake papaya halves at 350°F. for 15 minutes. Stuff with chicken mixture and serve with hot brown rice or barley. Yields 6 servings.

Creamy Potato Salad

 5 cups cubed boiled potatoes
 4 hard-cooked egg whites, chopped (discard yolks)
 2 tablespoons chopped pimiento
 2 tablespoons chopped green pepper
 4 ribs celery, diced
 2 tablespoons chopped onion
 2 tablespoons plain nonfat yogurt
 3 tablespoons no-oil Italian dressing
 1 tablespoon white vinegar
 2 teaspoons Hain no-salt prepared mustard
 ½ teaspoon dry mustard
 ½ teaspoon horseradish
 ⅛ teaspoon white pepper

Mix all ingredients well. Refrigerate for 1–2 hours, covered, allowing flavors to marry. Adjust seasoning to your taste. Yields 6–8 servings.

Summer Garden Antipasto*

1 10-oz. package frozen asparagus spears, or ¾ lb. fresh asparagus
2 cups sliced cucumbers
2 cups sliced mushrooms
1 cup no-oil Italian dressing
1 6½-oz. can water-packed white albacore tuna
   Crisp salad greens
2 cups cherry tomatoes

Cook asparagus in ½ cup water until barely tender; drain. Combine cucumbers, mushrooms, and asparagus in a 3-quart glass baking dish with a cover. Pour Italian dressing over the vegetables. Cover and refrigerate at least 1 hour. Drain tuna and remove bottom lid of can so you can push the tuna out in one piece. Place tuna in center of a large serving dish lined with crisp salad greens. Remove vegetables from the dressing, reserving dressing. Arrange the marinated vegetables and cherry tomatoes around the tuna. Pour dressing over the arrangement. Yields 8 servings.

For *Zucchini-Lettuce Salad* and *Cucumbers in Yogurt* recipes, see page 38.

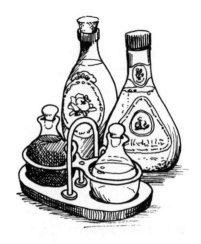

Salad Dressings

Italian Tomato Dressing

1 6-oz. can tomato paste
½ cup water
½ cup lemon juice
½ cup grated onion
1 clove garlic, crushed
1 teaspoon crushed basil leaves
1 teaspoon crushed oregano leaves

Combine all ingredients in a blender and mix well. Chill several hours or overnight. Before serving, shake well. Yields 2½ cups.

Garlic Dressing

1 cup plain nonfat yogurt
2 hard-cooked egg whites
½ cup fresh parsley

2 ribs celery, finely chopped

2 green onions, sliced

½ teaspoon fresh lemon juice

2 cloves garlic, crushed

Place all ingredients except yogurt in a blender or food processor and blend until chopped. Fold the mixture into the yogurt. Chill overnight in a covered container. Yields 1¼ cups.

Wine and Herb Dressing

1 cup wine vinegar

1 teaspoon crushed dried sweet basil (or 1½ teaspoons chopped fresh basil)

1 clove garlic

¼ teaspoon crushed dried rosemary (or ½ teaspoon chopped fresh rosemary)

¼ teaspoon crushed dried thyme (or ½ teaspoon chopped fresh thyme)

Combine all ingredients in a clean jar or bottle. Secure the lid. Let stand in refrigerator at least a week. The longer you allow mixture to stand, the better the flavors will marry. Yields 1 cup.

Zesty Mustard Dressing

For a good mustard flavor, combine dry mustard with an equal amount of cold water and stir until smooth. Let stand for 10 minutes. To vary the flavor, apple cider vinegar, white wine, or garlic may be added. Add to your favorite recipes: fish, sauces, casseroles, and salad dressings.

Yogurt Dressing

1 cup plain nonfat yogurt, thinned with nonfat milk to desired consistency

½ cup dry-curd or low-fat cottage cheese, mashed

2 tablespoons finely chopped cucumber

1 clove garlic, mashed

Mix all ingredients together and refrigerate at least 2 hours. Yields about 1¾ cups.

Zesty Sandwich Spread

1–2 teaspoons dry mustard

1–2 teaspoons water

1 cup plain nonfat yogurt

Combine dry mustard with equal amount of water. Let sit for 10 minutes. Stir mixture into yogurt. Good with tuna, chicken, potato salad, or coleslaw. Yields about 1 cup.

Seasoning Shaker #1

2 tablespoons crushed summer savory

1 tablespoon garlic powder

1¼ teaspoons ground cumin

1 teaspoon ground or crushed basil

1 teaspoon white pepper

1 teaspoon dry mustard

Combine all ingredients. Mix well and spoon into a shaker. Sprinkle on soup, salad, or any food that needs a taste booster.

Seasoning Shaker #2

1 tablespoon garlic powder

2 teaspoons onion powder

1 teaspoon marjoram

1 teaspoon ground or crushed basil

1 teaspoon dried parsley flakes

½ teaspoon celery seed

Combine ingredients. Mix well and spoon into a shaker.

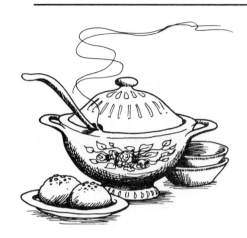

Soups

Seasoned Chicken Broth

3½ lbs. chicken parts, cut up, skinned, all visible fat removed

3½ quarts water

1 carrot, cut into coins

2 ribs celery, cut into pieces

1 large onion, cut in rings

1 leek, cleaned well and cut up

1 clove garlic, minced

1 medium bay leaf

½ teaspoon ground thyme

¼ teaspoon curry powder

⅛ teaspoon white pepper

Combine chicken, water, carrots, celery, onion, leek, and garlic in a large soup pot. Bring to a boil. Lower heat to simmer, cover, and cook for 2 hours. Remove chicken and strain the broth. Add the bay leaf, thyme, curry powder, and white pepper. Simmer uncovered for 1½ hours more. Remove bay leaf. Refrigerate overnight; remove fat that has hardened on top. Broth may be frozen in containers for future use. Yields about 2½ quarts.

Oriental Chicken Stock

12 cups water
3–4 lbs. chicken parts, skinned, all visible fat removed
2 whole scallions
2 tablespoons sherry (optional)
1 piece gingerroot, ½ inch thick

Bring water to a boil. Add all ingredients and return to a boil. Remove from heat and skim off the foam. Bring back to a boil. Simmer covered, with lid ajar, for 2–3 hours. Cool. Remove chicken and strain broth through a cheesecloth. Refrigerate overnight. Remove the fat that has hardened on top. May be frozen for later use. Yields 10 cups.

Velvet Chicken Soup

2 tablespoons sherry
1¼ teaspoon soy sauce
4 lightly beaten egg whites
3 medium size chicken breasts
8 cups clear chicken stock
1 10-oz. package frozen whole kernal corn, thawed
2 tablespoons cornstarch mixed with ¼ cup water
¼ teaspoon ground ginger

Combine 2 tablespoons sherry with ¼ teaspoon soy sauce and 2 of the beaten egg whites. Skin the chicken breasts, removing all visible fat. Cook and cut them into cubes. Add cubes to the egg-white mixture and set aside.

Heat chicken stock in a large saucepan. Add corn and bring to a boil. Add chicken mixture and stir in cornstarch mixture. Add the ginger and 1 teaspoon soy sauce. Turn heat off and slowly add remaining 2 egg whites. Stir in gently. Cool. Chill in refrigerator overnight. Heat to serve. Garnish with scallions. Yields 8 servings.

Barley and Mushroom Soup

6 cups Seasoned Chicken Broth (see page 189)
1 cup uncooked pearl barley
2 small potatoes, diced
2 medium onions, minced
2 carrots, grated
3 tablespoons chopped parsley
1 bay leaf
½ teaspoon celery seed
½ lb. mushrooms, sliced
2 parsnips, diced
1 cup nonfat skim milk
Dillweed

Cook barley in the chicken broth for 1 hour or until tender but not mushy. Add all other ingredients except mushrooms, parsnips, and milk. Add more broth if necessary. Cook covered over low heat for 45 minutes. Add mushrooms and parsnips 30 minutes before removing from heat. Discard bay leaf and stir in the skim milk. Reheat soup but do not let it boil. Garnish with dillweed. Yields 8 servings.

Beet Borscht

2 bunches of fresh beets
¼ cup raisins
1 6-oz. can apple juice concentrate, thawed
¼ cup apple cider vinegar
¼ cup lemon juice (or more to taste)
¼ teaspoon cloves
¼ teaspoon nutmeg
　Chopped green onion and/or cubed cucumber

Wash sand and dirt from beets under running water. Boil beets with enough water to cover, until slightly tender. Reserve the liquid; pour a little of it over the raisins to plump them. Cool beets and slip the skins off. Shred the beets and add to cooking liquid. Add the remaining ingredients and bring to a boil. Turn heat down and simmer slowly, covered, with lid slightly ajar, for 30 minutes until the flavors marry. Add more water if needed. Garnish with chopped green onions, cubed cucumber, or both. May be served hot or cold with boiled potatoes. Yields 10–12 generous servings.

Beet Borscht Odessa

1 large bunch of beets
2½ quarts water
1 6-oz. can apple juice concentrate, thawed
⅓ cup fresh lemon juice
1 large apple, grated
1 small onion, finely minced
1 tablespoon apple cider vinegar
⅛ teaspoon allspice

⅛ teaspoon cloves

1 tablespoon raisins (optional)

Boiled potatoes (optional)

Chopped green onions

Wash beets thoroughly and boil in 2½ quarts of water until tender. Remove beets, reserving liquid. Let cool. Slip skins off. In a soup pot, add apple juice concentrate, lemon juice, apple, onion, vinegar, and spices to the liquid. Bring to a boil. Lower heat and simmer, covered, for 30 minutes, allowing flavors to marry. Add more water if needed. Shred beets and add to liquid. Adjust seasoning. If too tart, add 1 tablespoon of raisins. Boiled potatoes may be added to borscht when ready to serve. Garnish with chopped green onions. Yields 10–12 servings.

Black Bean Soup

2 cups dried black beans

8 cups cold water

1 clove garlic, crushed

3 medium onions, chopped

2 stalks celery, sliced

2 bay leaves

2 tablespoons minced parsley

⅛ teaspoon white pepper

⅔ cup dry sherry (optional)

Soak beans overnight. Drain. In 8 cups cold water, cook beans over low heat until soft. In a nonstick skillet, sauté garlic, onions, and celery with 2 tablespoons of water from the soup kettle. Add the beans with the rest of the ingredients except the sherry. Continue cooking, covered, over low heat for 3 hours. Add a small amount of water if soup becomes too thick. Add sherry. Adjust seasoning to your taste. Remove bay leaves. Serve over hot barley or brown rice. Yields 6–8 servings.

Delicious Jellied Gazpacho

    1 envelope unflavored gelatin
    ½ cup water
    1 cup cold chicken broth
    ⅓ cup vinegar
    ½ teaspoon crushed basil
    ¼ teaspoon ground cloves
    ⅛ teaspoon Tabasco
       Dash of white pepper
  1½ cups finely chopped tomatoes
    ¼ cup finely chopped celery
    ¼ cup chopped zucchini
    ¼ cup finely chopped green or red pepper
    2 tablespoons finely chopped onion
    1 clove garlic, mashed in garlic press
       Mock Sour Kream (optional; see pages 56 and 225)

Sprinkle gelatin in ½ cup water to soften. In a saucepan, place over low heat and stir until gelatin is dissolved. Remove from heat. Add chicken broth, vinegar, and seasonings and mix together. Chill in refrigerator until consistency of unbeaten egg whites. Fold in tomatoes, celery, zucchini, green or red pepper, onion, and garlic. Cover and chill for 1 hour. Spoon into serving bowls and top each serving with a teaspoon of Mock Sour Kream if desired. Yields 8 servings.

Fish Stock

   5 lbs. fish bones and heads
2½ quarts water
  ½ cup sliced carrots
  2 large onions, sliced
  4 ribs celery, sliced
  1 teaspoon parsley
  1 bay leaf
 ⅛ teaspoon white pepper

Combine all ingredients in a large soup pot. Cover and simmer for 30 minutes. Allow to cool. Strain through cheesecloth. Discard the solids. Cover and refrigerate. Skim off the fat. May be frozen for future use. Yields approx. 2 quarts.

Fisherman's Chowder

 ¼ cup chopped onions
 ¼ cup chopped celery
 ¼ cup diced carrots
 1 tablespoon olive oil or nonstick cooking spray
 3 cloves garlic, minced
 4 bay leaves
 ½ teaspoon crushed oregano
 ⅛ teaspoon white pepper or to taste
4⅓ cups Fish Stock (see recipe above)
 1 lb. ripe tomatoes, peeled and chopped
 1 lb. mussels
 ¼ lb. scallops
 ¼ lb. clams

¼ cup chopped leeks

¾ cup dry white wine (optional)

2–4 tablespoons flour (whole-wheat, oat, rice, unbleached, or your choice)

Sauté onions, celery, and carrots in a nonstick skillet with olive oil or nonstick cooking spray for a few minutes. Add garlic, leeks, bay leaves, oregano, and pepper. Simmer for 5 minutes, then slowly bring to a boil. Set aside. Bring 4 cups of the fish stock to a boil in a large kettle. Add tomatoes, mussels, scallops, clams, and wine. Cook covered, with lid slightly ajar, over low heat for 10 minutes. Add sautéed vegetables. Stir lightly until well mixed. Add 2 tablespoons flour to remaining ⅓ cup fish stock; stir to form a paste. Stir flour mixture into the soup. Simmer and continue stirring to keep lumps from forming as the soup thickens. If necessary, repeat this procedure until desired thickness is achieved. Remove bay leaf. Yields 8 servings.

Edythe's Fresh Vegetable Soup*

4 cups Seasoned Chicken Broth (see page 189) or water

3 cloves garlic, minced

1 medium zucchini, sliced

1 turnip, diced

1 10-oz. package frozen corn kernels

2 large onions, chopped

1 cup diced carrots

1 cup cut-up broccoli

1 small eggplant, peeled and cubed

1 16-oz. can unsalted tomatoes, mashed

½ teaspoon ground coriander

⅛ teaspoon white pepper

1 bay leaf

1 teaspoon basil

½ cup whole-wheat elbow macaroni, cooked and drained[1]

In a soup pot, bring chicken broth or water to a boil. Reduce heat. Add all remaining ingredients except macaroni. Bring back to a boil. Reduce to simmer and simmer, with lid slightly ajar, 10 minutes or until vegetables are barely tender. Add macaroni and simmer 5 minutes longer. Remove bay leaf. Yields 6 servings.

[1] Do not use any macaroni on Soup Day during Jump-Start. Macaroni adds calories to this soup.

Gazpacho*

1 quart no-salt-added tomato juice or no-salt-added V8 juice, chilled

2 tablespoons wine vinegar

1 clove garlic

½ green pepper, cut in pieces

1 medium zucchini

1 rib celery, cut in pieces

2 ripe tomatoes

½ small onion

½ teaspoon dried basil

¼ teaspoon white pepper

3 teaspoons chopped parsley

Use the chopping blade in the bowl of your food processor. Start with 2 cups of tomato juice. Add remaining ingredients and process until well blended. Add 1 more cup of tomato juice and process until well blended. Pour the remaining tomato juice and the blended mixture into a 1½-quart container. Stir. Chill for several hours. If you are in a hurry to serve, pour into serving dishes with an ice cube in each dish. Garnish with chopped parsley. Yields 6 (8-oz.) servings.

Lentil–Sweet Potato Soup

  7 cups chicken stock, no-salt-added tomato juice, or water
  1 16-oz. package of lentils
4–6 carrots, cut in coins
  1 large sweet potato, peeled and cubed
  1 large onion, diced
  3 ribs celery, diced
  2 cloves garlic, minced
  1 large bay leaf
  ½ teaspoon marjoram
  ¼ teaspoon allspice
    Chopped parsley

In a large soup kettle, combine liquid and lentils. Bring to a boil. Cover and cook over low heat for 1–1½ hours. Add vegetables, garlic, bay leaf, and marjoram. Simmer covered for 45 minutes. Add allspice and cook 5 minutes longer. For a thicker soup, simmer for 20–30 minutes uncovered. Remove bay leaf. Garnish with chopped parsley. Serve over cooked barley or brown rice. Yields 10–12 servings.

Split-Pea Soup

  1 lb. green split peas
2½ quarts water or chicken stock
  1 large onion, diced

2 cloves garlic, minced
1 bay leaf
½ teaspoon thyme
4 carrots, cut into small pieces
3 ribs celery, chopped
3 tablespoons chopped parsley
1 tablespoon Angostura bitters (optional)
  Sliced mushrooms (optional)
  Grated carrot (optional)

Wash peas thoroughly. Cover peas with water and soak overnight. Drain. Add 2½ quarts water or chicken stock, onion, garlic, bay leaf, and thyme. Bring to a boil. Cover and simmer for 2 hours, stirring occasionally. Add carrot pieces, celery, and parsley. Cover and cook slowly for 1 hour and 45 minutes. Remove bay leaf and press entire mixture through a sieve, or put half the peas in a blender and blend. Return peas to the pot. Add mushrooms and/or grated carrots if desired; stir and heat. (For thicker soup, simmer uncovered for 20–30 minutes.) Just before serving, stir in Angostura bitters if desired. Good served with cooked brown rice or cooked garbanzos (chick-peas). Yields 8–10 servings.

Mexican Split-Pea Soup

1 lb. split peas
2½ quarts water or chicken stock
1 16-oz. can unsalted tomatoes
4 carrots, cut in small pieces
1 large onion, diced
2 celery ribs, diced
1 clove garlic, minced
1 bay leaf

½ teaspoon crushed oregano

½ teaspoon dry mustard

1 teaspoon cumino seeds, crushed with a mortar and pestle (or use ground cumin)

1 teaspoon chopped cilantro

Sliced fresh mushrooms (optional)

Grated carrot (optional)

Wash peas thoroughly. Soak overnight in enough water to cover. Drain; save the water. Add enough water or chicken stock to the soaking water to make 2½ quarts. Place all ingredients except mushrooms and grated carrot in a soup pot and bring to a boil. Reduce heat and simmer, covered, for 1½–2 hours. Remove bay leaf. Press entire mixture through a sieve, or put half the mixture in a blender and blend. Return to pot, adding sliced mushrooms and/or grated carrot if desired. Stir and heat. Adjust thickness to your liking by adding liquid or, for thicker soup, simmer uncovered for 20–30 minutes. Good served with hot brown rice or cooked garbanzos (chick-peas). Yields 8–10 servings.

Okra Gumbo

1 lb. okra

2 tablespoons water

2 large onions, diced

3 celery ribs, sliced, including leaves

½ cup chopped green pepper

2 cloves garlic, minced

5 cups water

1 cup unsalted tomatoes, mashed

¼ teaspoon oregano

1 bay leaf

¼ lb. white-meat fish, cubed (optional)

2 cups cooked brown rice

Cut off the ends of the okra and slice into ½-inch pieces. In a nonstick skillet, heat 2 tablespoons water and stir in okra, onions, celery, green pepper, and garlic. Sauté for 5 minutes, stirring to prevent sticking. Add 5 cups water, tomatoes, oregano, and bay leaf. Cover and simmer slowly for 45 minutes to 1 hour. Add fish 30 minutes before end of cooking time. Remove bay leaf. Serve over hot brown rice. Yields 6–8 servings.

Tuna Vegetable Soup

1 medium onion, chopped

4 celery ribs, sliced

3 carrots, sliced in coins

1 green pepper, cut in small pieces

2 tablespoons chicken broth or water

1 16-oz. can tomatoes, slightly mashed

8 cups chicken broth

1½ teaspoons summer savory

1 teaspoon sweet basil

1 bay leaf

1 6½-oz. can water-packed, low-sodium tuna, drained

1 cup cooked brown rice

In a nonstick skillet, sauté onion, celery, carrots, and green pepper in 2 tablespoons chicken broth or water. In a soup pot, stir in tomatoes, 8 cups chicken broth, summer savory, sweet basil, and bay leaf. Simmer, covered, for 25 minutes. Stir in tuna and rice; simmer 5 minutes. Remove bay leaf. Yields 8 servings.

Chili

1 lb. dried red kidney beans

1 16-oz. can unsalted tomatoes, chopped

2 fresh tomatoes, skinned and chopped

1 6-oz. can tomato paste

3 tablespoons cumino seeds, crushed with a mortar and pestle (or use 3 teaspoons ground cumin)

3 cloves garlic, minced

3 medium onions, chopped

3 tablespoons chili powder

2 tablespoons picante sauce (mild or hot)

¼ teaspoon crushed oregano

2 tablespoons sherry (optional)

Wash beans well and soak overnight in enough water to allow for the beans to double in bulk. Do not drain. Bring beans to a boil. Cover and simmer while preparing the other ingredients. Add canned and fresh tomatoes, tomato paste, and cumino seeds and bring to a boil. Lower the heat. Add the remaining ingredients except sherry. Cover and cook over low heat for 2 hours or until beans are soft, stirring occasionally. Add more water if the mixture becomes too thick. Add sherry just before removing from the heat. Adjust seasoning to your liking. Yields 6–8 servings.

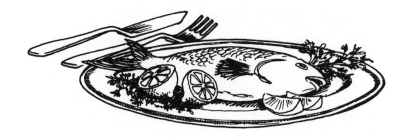

Fish

Basic Broiled Fish*

Rinse fish quickly in cold water and pat dry with a paper towel. Squeeze a generous amount of lemon juice on fish 20–30 minutes before broiling. Preheat broiling pan for at least 10 minutes to broiling heat (approx. 550°F.). Place fish on preheated broiling rack. Broil fillets and steaks 2 inches from flame; broil split fish and whole dressed fish 2–6 inches from flame. Broil about 20 minutes per inch of thickness at the thickest part of the fish. (A good average thickness for fillets is 1 inch.)

Baked Flounder*

Place rinsed fish in a glass baking dish. Mix ⅓ cup white wine, 1 tablespoon chopped parsley, and 2 teaspoons lemon juice. Pour mixture over the fish. Bake uncovered at 425°F. for 12–15 minutes or until fish flakes with a fork.

Broiled Sole Fillets*

For extra good flavor, squeeze lemon juice on fish about 15–20 minutes before broiling. Baste fillets with mashed garlic and lemon juice. Broil for 10–12 minutes or until fish flakes with a fork. Broil thin fillets very near the flame to brown quickly.

Baked Halibut*

Place halibut in a glass baking dish. Combine ¼ cup dry white wine with 1 tablespoon lemon juice and pour over the fish. Bake uncovered at 350°F. for 25–30 minutes or until fish flakes with a fork. Sprinkle with chopped parsley about 4–5 minutes before serving.

Salmon is also good baked this way. If possible, use the tail end of the salmon—it is meatier and has fewer small bones.

Baked Fish Supreme

- 4 lbs. fish (halibut, red snapper, hake, or your favorite fish)
- ½ teaspoon lemon juice
- 2 tablespoons dry mustard
- 2 tablespoons red horseradish
- 1 2-oz. jar of capers, drained (optional)
- 1 cup plain nonfat yogurt
- ½ teaspoon grated sapsago cheese (optional)

Preheat oven to 350°F. Place fish in a shallow baking dish. Sprinkle with lemon juice. Dot with mustard, horseradish, and capers. Smooth yogurt over fish and sprinkle the sapsago cheese on top. Bake uncovered in preheated 350°F. oven for 20 minutes. May be prepared in advance and refrigerated before cooking. Yields 4–6 servings.

Baked Fish, Complete Dish

4 lbs. filleted red snapper or white fish, cut into serving pieces
2 12-oz. cans no-salt-added tomato juice
2 cups plain nonfat yogurt
1 10-oz. package frozen mixed vegetables
3 medium-size potatoes, cut into small pieces
2 carrots, cut into small pieces
3 celery ribs, cut into small pieces
2 tablespoons minced onion
   Dillweed

Combine all ingredients except dillweed. Marinate in refrigerator, covered, overnight. Strain the liquid off and set aside. Put the vegetables in the bottom of a baking dish. Place the fish on top and sprinkle a little dillweed over the fish. Pour in reserved marinade. Cover with foil. Bake in a 350°F. oven for 20 minutes. Remove foil and continue to bake for 30 minutes more. Yields 4–6 servings.

Baked Snapper Fillets

Preheat oven to 375°F. Baste red snapper fillets with no-salt-added V8 juice and lemon juice. Sprinkle with dillweed. Allow to stand in baking dish for 10 minutes. Place fish in preheated 375°F. oven and bake 20–25 minutes or until fish flakes with a fork. Serve with colorful vegetables.

Gefilte Fish

      7 yellow onions, 3 sliced and 4 to grind with fish (reserve
         the skins)
      5 carrots, sliced into coins
   7½ cups water
      ½ cup apple juice concentrate, thawed
      6 lbs. fish of your choice, filleted (ask for fishhead and
         bones at your market)
      6 egg whites, well beaten
   1½ teaspoons white pepper
   1½ cups matzo meal (approx.)
   1⅓ cups ice water (approx.)
         Carrots
         Parsley

Wash onion skins. Place them in bottom of soup pot. Combine the 3 sliced onions and the sliced carrots with 7½ cups water, apple juice concentrate, fish bones and head. Cook over medium heat while preparing the fish. Put the fish and 4 onions through food grinder, twice. Place fish and onions in a chopping bowl. Add egg whites and pepper. Add matzo meal ½ cup at a time, alternating with ice water ⅓ cup at a time. Chop until very fine (this makes the fish fluffy). Moisten your hands and shape mixture into balls. Gently lay fish-balls in the simmering stock. Cover, leaving the lid ajar, and cook over low heat for 1 hour. Remove cover and continue to cook over low heat for 30 minutes. Cool the fish slightly before removing to a platter. Strain the stock and freeze for future use; fish may also be frozen. Arrange cooked carrot coins and parsley around the fish. Serve with horseradish. Yields 24 medium pieces.

Tuna or Zucchini Lasagna

 1 28-oz. can unsalted tomatoes

 2 6-oz. cans tomato paste

 1 6-oz. can unsalted tomato sauce

 1 large onion, chopped

½ cup chopped green pepper

 2 cloves garlic, minced

2½ teaspoons no-salt Italian seasoning

 2 6½-oz. cans water-packed tuna, drained, or 4 large zucchini, sliced lengthwise

½ lb. mushrooms, sliced

 1 8-oz. package whole-wheat lasagna noodles, cooked
Cheese mixture (see below)

Combine first seven ingredients in a large kettle and bring to a boil. Reduce heat. Cover and simmer for 15 minutes. Fold in the tuna (or zucchini) and mushrooms. Pour 1 cup of sauce into a shallow 3-quart baking dish. Layer one-third of the noodles lengthwise over the sauce. Pour 1¼ cups sauce over the noodles. Top with cheese mixture. Repeat layers until all of the ingredients are used up. Reserve enough sauce to top the lasagna last. Bake lasagne uncovered at 350°F. for 1 hour. Let stand about 10 minutes before slicing. Yields 8–10 servings.

Cheese Mixture for Lasagna

1 lb. dry-curd cottage cheese or hoop cheese, mashed smooth

¼ cup grated sapsago cheese

½ cup low-fat buttermilk

4 egg whites, stiffly beaten

Combine cottage cheese, sapsago cheese, and buttermilk. Fold in beaten egg whites.

Salmon-Stuffed Cabbage Rolls

1 medium cabbage

½ cup chopped green pepper

½ cup chopped onion

2 tablespoons olive oil or water, or nonstick cooking spray

1 cup cooked brown rice

3 egg whites, slightly beaten

1 15½-oz. can pink salmon, drained and crumbled (including bones)

1 teaspoon sweet basil

1 15-oz. can unsalted tomato sauce

1 16-oz. can unsalted tomatoes

½ teaspoon caraway seeds

Remove core from the cabbage. Place cabbage, core side down, in pot of boiling water. Remove and drain the leaves as they begin to separate. Sauté the green pepper and onion in olive oil or water in a nonstick skillet until soft. Combine rice, egg whites, salmon, and basil with sautéed vegetables. Spoon the mixture onto cabbage leaves. Roll up leaves, securing the filling by tucking in the sides. Line a 3-quart casserole dish with other cabbage leaves. Lay cabbage rolls on top. Combine tomato sauce with undrained tomatoes and pour over the cabbage rolls. Sprinkle with caraway seeds. Cover and bake at 350°F. for 45 minutes. Remove cover and bake for 30 minutes longer. Yields 6–8 servings.

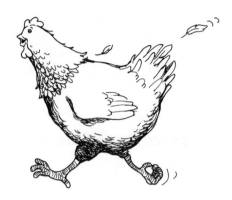

Poultry

Sloppy Joes

- 1 teaspoon dry mustard
- 3 tablespoons + 1 teaspoon apple juice concentrate, thawed
- 1 lb. ground turkey
- ½ cup chopped green pepper
- ½ cup chopped onion
- 2 cloves garlic, minced
- 3¼ cups canned unsalted tomatoes, cut up
- 1 6-oz. can tomato paste
- 3 tablespoons apple cider vinegar
- 8 Pritikin English Muffins (found in frozen-food case), or wheat pita rounds

Combine mustard and 1 teaspoon apple juice concentrate. Let stand for 10 minutes. Brown ground turkey with green pepper, onion, and garlic in a large nonstick skillet. Stir to crumble the meat. Pour off any fat that has drained from the meat. Stir in tomatoes, tomato paste, 3 tablespoons apple juice concentrate, vinegar, and mustard mixture. Simmer uncovered for 30 minutes, stirring occasionally. Split English muffins and toast lightly. Serve Sloppy Joe mixture on muffins, or in whole-wheat pita rounds. Yields 8 servings.

Baked Bar-B-Que Chicken

- 1 cup water
- ¼ cup vinegar
- 1 6-oz. can tomato paste
- ¼ cup apple juice concentrate, thawed, or ½ cup sugar-free applesauce
- 1 tablespoon chili powder
- 1 teaspoon dry mustard
- ¼ teaspoon garlic powder
- 3 lbs. chicken breasts, skinned, all visible fat removed

Combine water, vinegar, tomato paste, apple juice concentrate, chili powder, dry mustard, and garlic powder in a medium-size saucepan, stirring to blend. Simmer for 10 minutes. Arrange chicken in a shallow baking pan. Pour sauce over chicken to cover evenly. Bake at 350°F. for 1 hour and 15 minutes. Yields 5–6 servings.

Vegetables with Noodles and Chicken

- 4 chicken breasts, skinned, boned, all visible fat removed
- 2 tablespoons chicken broth or water
- 4 large tomatoes, chopped
- 2 cups thinly sliced mushrooms
- 1½ cups thinly sliced zucchini
- ¼ cup thinly sliced green onions

½ teaspoon crushed basil
Dash of white pepper
½ lb. whole-grain medium noodles

With a mallet or side of meat cleaver, flatten chicken breasts. In medium nonstick skillet over low heat, sauté chicken breasts in chicken broth, covered, about 20–25 minutes. While chicken breasts are cooking, place tomatoes in saucepan, cover, and cook over low heat until tender, about 10 minutes. Add mushrooms, zucchini, green onions, basil, and pepper. Cover and cook 5 minutes. Remove cover and cook 10 minutes longer to reduce some of the liquid. Add noodles to 3 quarts boiling water slowly so that water continues to boil. Stir occasionally. Cook uncovered about 8 minutes or until tender. Drain noodles and arrange on a large serving dish. Top with chicken breasts and spoon vegetable mixture on top. Yields 4 servings.

Chicken and Mushrooms

1 lb. fresh mushrooms, sliced
½ cup minced onion, divided
½ cup diced green pepper
1 clove garlic, minced
2 tablespoons water or olive oil
1 16-oz. can unsalted tomatoes, chopped
1 teaspoon oregano
¼ teaspoon white pepper
4 cups diced cooked chicken breast, skinned, all visible fat removed

In a nonstick skillet, sauté mushrooms, half the onion, green pepper, and garlic in water or olive oil for 4–5 minutes. Stir in rest of onion, tomatoes, and seasonings. Bring to a boil. Reduce heat and simmer uncovered for 10 minutes. Add chicken. Heat until chicken is hot. Serve in a brown rice ring. Yields 6–8 servings.

Chicken and Orange Sauce*

6 chicken breasts, skinned, all visible fat removed
1 cup sliced mushrooms
½ cup fresh-squeezed orange juice
1 teaspoon grated orange rind
½ cup chicken stock
1 scant teaspoon ground ginger
1 tablespoon low-salt soy sauce
½ cup water
2 tablespoons cornstarch
3 tablespoons finely chopped parsley

Arrange chicken breasts in a glass baking dish. Place sliced mushrooms over chicken. Combine orange juice, orange rind, chicken stock, ginger, soy sauce, and water. Pour over chicken and mushrooms. Bake at 350°F. for 45 minutes. Remove from oven, baste the chicken and mushrooms with liquid from baking dish. Remove the chicken and mushrooms from the baking dish; keep them warm. In a saucepan, combine cornstarch with the remaining juices. Heat and stir until sauce is thickened. Pour over chicken and mushrooms. If desired, serve over fluffy brown rice or bulgur wheat.[1] Garnish with chopped parsley. Yields 6 servings.

[1] In the Jump-Start phase, serve with vegetables instead of brown rice or bulgur wheat.

Boneless Breast of Chicken with Orange and Parsley Sauce*

1½ lbs. chicken breasts, boned, skinned, all visible fat removed

1 bunch green onions with stems, chopped

1 medium green pepper, chopped

½ cup Zante currants (small white raisins)

¼ cup lemon juice

½ teaspoon ground ginger

½ teaspoon ground cloves

¼ teaspoon allspice

1 tablespoon soy sauce

½ lb. mushrooms, sliced

4 tablespoons cornstarch

½ cup water

2 medium oranges, sectioned

1 cup seedless grapes

½ cup chopped parsley

> Brown chicken breasts under broiler. In a nonstick skillet, combine onions, green pepper, currants, lemon juice, spices, soy sauce, and chicken. Cover and cook over medium heat for a few minutes. Add mushrooms. Mix cornstarch with ½ cup water and stir into chicken mixture. Stir until thick. Add oranges, grapes, and parsley. Heat for a few minutes and serve over hot brown rice.[1] Yields 6 servings.

[1] In Jump-Start, serve over vegetables instead of rice.

Broiled Chicken Breasts*

½ cup dry white wine or water

¼ cup soy sauce, diluted with ¼ cup water

3 cloves garlic, finely minced

2 fingers fresh gingerroot, finely minced

8 chicken breasts, skinned, all visible fat removed

Combine wine or water, diluted soy sauce, garlic, and ginger. Marinate chicken breasts in mixture for at least 2 hours, covered in the refrigerator. Marinate longer if possible. Broil chicken, 6 inches from heat, basting often with the marinade, for 20 minutes. Turn and continue broiling and basting 20 minutes longer. May be served hot or cold. Yields 8 servings.

Mexican Chicken

6 chicken breasts, skinned, with all visible fat removed

½ cup Seasoned Chicken Broth (see page 189)

1 teaspoon chopped cilantro

1 teaspoon ground cumin

6–8 cups chili (see pages 202 and 235)

Simmer chicken breasts in chicken broth, cilantro, and ground cumin for 10 minutes. Set aside. Place chili in a food processor. Process until a sauce is formed. If too thick, add water or chicken broth. Pour over chicken breasts and allow to simmer for 30–40 minutes or until the chicken is tender. Remove chicken to a platter and spoon the sauce over the chicken. Good with hot brown rice or spaghetti. Yields 6 servings.

Variation: Place chicken and processed chili in a baking dish and bake, covered, at 350°F. for 15 minutes. Remove lid and allow to brown for 15 minutes more. Baste chicken with chili.

¹ Chili can be made a day or two in advance.

Chicken Cacciatore

4–6 chicken breast halves, skinned, all visible fat removed
¼ cup chicken broth
¼ cup water
1 large green pepper, thinly sliced
2 large onions, thinly sliced
1 16-oz. can unsalted tomatoes
1 6-oz. can tomato paste
¾ cup dry red wine
1 teaspoon oregano leaves
2 cloves garlic, minced
¼ teaspoon white pepper

Brown chicken under broiler flame. In a Dutch oven–type pot, heat chicken broth and ¼ cup water. Add chicken, green pepper, and onions. Cover and cook about 5 minutes. Add tomatoes, tomato paste, wine, oregano, garlic, and pepper. Cover and cook over low heat, stirring occasionally. Simmer for 45 minutes. Serve with whole-wheat thin spaghetti or wheat-free corn pasta. Yields 4–6 servings.

Chicken Chop Suey

  2 chicken breasts, boned, skinned, and halved, all visible
     fat removed
  1 cup chicken broth
  ¼ cup soy sauce
  ½ teaspoon ground ginger
  3 ribs celery, sliced
  1 8-oz. can water chestnuts, drained and sliced
  1 medium onion, halved and sliced
  1 cup sliced fresh mushrooms
  2 tablespoons bean sprouts

Cut chicken into strips 2 inches long and ½ inch thick.
Place in a nonstick skillet. Add chicken broth, soy sauce,
ginger, celery, water chestnuts, and onion. Cover and
cook over low heat for 30 minutes. Add mushrooms
and bean sprouts. Cover and cook over medium heat
for 15 minutes. Serve over brown rice or spoon-size
shredded wheat. Yields 4–6 servings.

Chicken Breasts and Mushroom Sauce*

4–5 chicken breasts, halved, boned, skinned, all visible fat
     removed
  1 cup chicken broth
  ¼ cup Sauterne wine
  1 tablespoon tomato paste
  1 clove garlic, minced
  2 tablespoons minced onion
  1 tablespoon soy sauce
  1 teaspoon dry mustard

2 tablespoons cornstarch

2 tablespoons water

½ lb. fresh mushrooms, sliced

Place chicken breasts in a nonstick skillet. Combine chicken broth, wine, tomato paste, garlic, onion, soy sauce, and mustard, and pour over the chicken. Cover and cook over low heat for 30 minutes. Dissolve cornstarch in 2 tablespoons water. Stir into skillet. Add mushrooms and continue cooking over low heat for 30 minutes. Yields 4–5 servings.

Hawaiian Chicken

6 chicken breasts, skinned, all visible fat removed

1 bunch green onions, finely sliced

1 cup finely sliced green pepper

½ cup currants

¼ cup fresh lemon juice

1 tablespoon soy sauce

½ teaspoon ginger

½ teaspoon ground cloves

¼ teaspoon allspice

1 8-oz. can water chestnuts, drained and sliced

½ lb. mushrooms, sliced

3 tablespoons cornstarch

½ cup water

2 oranges, sectioned

½ cup seedless grapes

½ cup finely chopped fresh parsley

Brown chicken under broiler. Transfer to a large nonstick skillet. Over medium heat, add onions, green pepper, currants, lemon juice, soy sauce, and spices. Cover and cook about 2–3 minutes. Stir and replace cover, reduce heat, and simmer for 45 minutes. Add water chestnuts and mushrooms. Dissolve cornstarch in ½ cup water. Add to chicken mixture and stir until thickened. Add orange sections, grapes, and parsley. Stir until completely heated. Serve over brown rice. Yields 6 servings.

Chicken 'n' Rice

5–6 chicken breasts, skinned, all visible fat removed
  1 large onion, thinly sliced
  3 tablespoons chicken broth or no-salt-added tomato juice
  3 cups canned unsalted tomatoes
  1 clove garlic, crushed
  1 small bay leaf
  ⅛ teaspoon white pepper
  1 cup brown rice, washed and drained
    Pimiento strips
    Green pepper rings

Brown chicken breasts under broiler. Sauté onion in chicken broth or tomato juice. Place chicken over onions in ovenproof casserole dish with a lid. Heat tomatoes to boiling point and add to chicken, with garlic, bay leaf, and pepper. Add rice. Cook covered in a 350°F. oven. Remove lid and stir rice after 15 minutes. Replace lid and continue cooking until rice is tender and fluffy and all liquid is absorbed (about 1 hour total cooking time). Turn onto a warm serving platter. Discard the bay leaf. Garnish with pimiento strips and green pepper rings. Yields 5–6 servings.

Steamed Chicken Dinner

Juice of 1½ medium lemons
3 teaspoons crushed sweet basil
2 bay leaves, crushed
1 lb. chicken breasts, skinned, all visible fat removed
4 medium carrots, sliced into 2-inch lengths
3 medium potatoes, peeled and sliced thin
⅛ teaspoon white pepper
Chopped parsley

Pour water into a 6- or 7-quart steamer pot, making sure that no water reaches up to the bottom of the steamer basket. Bring water to a boil. Add juice of ½ lemon, half of the basil, and crushed bay leaves. Arrange chicken breasts in steamer basket. Cover and steam for 10 minutes. Add carrots and potatoes. Add the remaining lemon juice and sprinkle with the remaining basil and white pepper. Cover and steam for 20 minutes, or until potatoes and carrots are tender and the chicken is done. Place chicken on a serving dish and arrange vegetables around it. Spoon some of the cooking liquid over the top. Garnish with chopped parsley. Yields 4–5 servings.

Chicken Broccoli Casserole

5 cups water
5–6 breasts of chicken, skinned, all visible fat removed
2 ribs celery, cut into large pieces
1 large carrot
1 medium onion
½ cup flour

¾ cup nonfat skim milk

2 cups chicken broth, reserved from boiling the chicken

⅛ teaspoon white pepper

½ teaspoon curry powder

1 cup Mock Sour Kream (see pages 56 and 225)

1 teaspoon fresh lemon or lime juice

1½ lbs. fresh broccoli or 2 10-oz. packages frozen

2 cups bread crumbs

Bring 5 cups water to a boil. Add chicken, celery, carrot, and onion. Reduce heat to simmer and cook until chicken is tender, about 45 minutes. (This may be done the day before.) Remove the chicken and strain the broth; discard cooked vegetables; reserve the broth. Cube the chicken and set aside. To prepare the sauce, blend flour and milk until smooth. Add 2 cups of the reserved chicken broth; cook and stir until thickened. Add pepper and curry powder. Remove from heat and add the Mock Sour Kream and lemon juice. Steam broccoli until just barely tender. Cut into pieces and place in a shallow baking dish. Top with chicken, sauce, and bread crumbs. Bake at 350°F. about 45 minutes. Serve over hot barley or pasta. Yields about 6 generous servings.

Chicken in Foil

This is a perfect meal to ''brown bag.'' Preheat oven to 325°F. Make an individual foil package for each serving. On each piece of foil, place one or two chicken breasts with all skin and visible fat removed, one potato that has been peeled and cut into thin wedges, and two carrots that have been cut into coins. Sprinkle with white pepper and chopped parsley or any of your favorite seasonings. Fold to seal foil securely. Bake in a preheated 325°F. oven for 1 hour.

Cranberry Apple Stuffing

1 medium chopped onion
1½ cups chopped celery
½ cup + 2 tablespoons Seasoned Chicken Broth (see page 189)
4 cups day-old cubed sourdough bread
2 cups pared and sliced apples
1 cup fresh chopped cranberries
¼ teaspoon crushed thyme
¼ teaspoon rosemary
¼ teaspoon marjoram
⅛ teaspoon white pepper

Sauté onion and celery in 2 tablespoons chicken broth until tender. In a large bowl combine all the ingredients. Toss lightly to mix. Good as poultry stuffing or to eat as a separate side dish. Yields 6 servings.

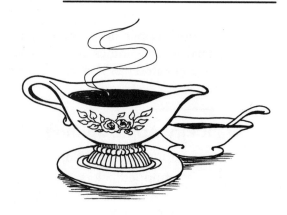

Sauces and Marinades

Marinade Sauce Oriental for Flank Steak or Chicken Breasts

- 3 tablespoons chopped onion
- 1 tablespoon diced green pepper
- 2 tablespoons water
- 1 tablespoon low-salt soy sauce
- 1 clove garlic, mashed
- 2 tablespoons grated orange peel
- 1 teaspoon ground ginger
- ½ cup sherry

Sauté onion and green pepper in 2 tablespoons water. Add the rest of the ingredients and simmer covered for 5 minutes. Cool. To use marinade, pour over flank steak or chicken that has been scored. Allow to marinate several hours, covered in refrigerator. Remove meat from marinade. For flank steak, broil 3 inches from heat, brushing with marinade. Turn once after 8–10 minutes or until cooked to desired doneness. Cut steak diagonally to serve. For chicken, brush chicken with sauce and broil 6 inches from heat for 5 minutes. Turn, brush with sauce, and broil 3 minutes. (Use all the sauce.) Yields enough marinade for 1½ lbs. flank steak or 1½ lbs. chicken breasts (use boneless chicken breasts, skinned, all visible fat removed).

Spicy Marinade for Flank Steak or Chicken

3 teaspoons dry mustard
2 tablespoons vinegar
2 tablespoons picante sauce
3 teaspoons garlic powder
1 tablespoon lemon juice

Mix all ingredients together. Pour over scored flank steak or chicken and allow meat to marinate several hours or overnight, covered and refrigerated. Turn steak to evenly coat with marinade. Follow instructions for cooking from Marinade Sauce Oriental recipe on page 222. Yields enough sauce for 1½ lbs. steak or 1½ lbs. boneless chicken breasts (skinned, all visible fat removed).

Sherry Chicken Marinade

2 teaspoons low-salt soy sauce diluted with 2 teaspoons water
1 tablespoon dry sherry
¼ teaspoon ground ginger
1 lb. boneless chicken breasts, skinned, all visible fat removed, cut into thin strips
1 cup chicken broth
1 tablespoon cornstarch

3 cups hot cooked brown rice

3 tablespoons diced pimiento

Green and red pepper strips

Combine water-diluted soy sauce, sherry, and ginger. Add chicken strips to marinade. Refrigerate for several hours or overnight, covered. In a large nonstick skillet, add chicken and ¾ cup chicken broth. Cook over medium heat, stirring, for about 5 minutes. Mix remaining ¼ cup broth with cornstarch. Add to chicken; cook and stir until mixture has thickened. Mix the pimiento and hot rice together. Pour chicken mixture over a bed of the rice mixture. Garnish with green and red pepper strips. Yields about 6 servings.

Cranberry Sauce

1 6-oz. can apple juice concentrate, thawed

2 oz. water

3 cups fresh cranberries, rinsed and drained

Combine apple juice concentrate and water in a saucepan. Bring to a boil. Add cranberries and continue to boil for 7–10 minutes uncovered, stirring occasionally. Remove from heat. May be served warm or cold. Yields 4 servings.

Karen's Fresh Tomato Sauce

1 onion, sliced

3–4 cloves garlic, crushed

2 tablespoons olive oil

4–6 Roma tomatoes or vine-ripened tomatoes, peeled and quartered

¼–⅓ cup fresh basil

Fresh oregano to taste

Pepper to taste

Sauté onion and garlic in olive oil. Add remaining ingredients and simmer 20–30 minutes to desired tenderness. Serve over pasta. Yields 2 servings.

Mock Sour Kream*

1 cup dry-curd or low-fat cottage cheese

¼ cup nonfat skim milk

½ teaspoon fresh lemon juice

Combine ingredients in a blender and blend until smooth. If consistency is too thick, add more milk a teaspoon at a time until desired thickness is achieved. Use for dips. Mix your own blend of herbs and spices. Season with chives or onions and serve over baked potatoes. Yields approx. 1½ cups.

Angostura Yogurt Sauce

1 cup plain nonfat yogurt

¼ teaspoon Angostura bitters

Combine the yogurt and Angostura. Mix thoroughly. Refrigerate at least 1 hour before serving. Good over fruit. Yields 1 cup.

Mushroom Marinade

3 tablespoons lemon juice

3 tablespoons water

1 bay leaf

1 cup mushrooms, cleaned and halved
½ teaspoon tarragon
2 tablespoons minced parsley

Bring lemon juice, water, and bay leaf to a boil, then add mushrooms and tarragon. Cover and simmer until mushrooms are barely cooked. Cool in liquid, then drain and toss mushrooms with parsley. Refrigerate for several hours or overnight. Great as a side dish or as an appetizer. Yields 4 servings.

Tomato Ketchup

½ cup chopped onions
3 cloves garlic, minced
2 tablespoons water
1 16-oz. can unsalted tomatoes
1 15-oz. can no-salt-added tomato sauce
1 6-oz. can tomato paste
½ cup apple cider vinegar
1 teaspoon crushed basil leaves
1 teaspoon crushed rosemary leaves
1 teaspoon crushed oregano leaves

In a 3-quart saucepan, cook onions and garlic in 2 tablespoons water 2–3 minutes, until onion is soft. Add tomatoes and mash with a fork. Stir in remaining ingredients. Bring to a boil, reduce heat to simmer, and cook until mixture is desired thickness and flavors are blended. Cool and refrigerate. May be frozen indefinitely. To use as a sauce, dilute with water or unsalted tomato juice. Yields 3–3½ cups.

Homemade Picante Sauce*

3 large tomatoes, cubed
1 6-oz. can tomato puree
¼ teaspoon minced garlic
3 tablespoons fresh cilantro
3 whole green chiles (not jalapeños)

Combine ingredients in food processor and process until chunky. Store in refrigerator. Yields 1 cup.

Marinara Sauce*

2 tablespoons extra-virgin olive oil[1]
3 cups chopped onions
4 cloves garlic, chopped
2 cups diced carrots (about 5 or 6)
6 cups chopped fresh tomatoes (or canned, drained well)[2]
4 tablespoons dried basil, or 3 tablespoons fresh basil
White pepper to taste
Water

Heat oil in a large saucepan or skillet; add onions, garlic, and carrots. Sauté until onions begin to brown. Add tomatoes, basil, and white pepper. Cover and simmer 15 minutes. Pour sauce into food processor or blender 2 cups at a time and puree to a creamy consistency. Return to pan and stir in water ¼ cup at a time until desired consistency. Cover and simmer for 10 minutes. Yields 6 servings.

[1] Omit olive oil during Jump-Start phase and sauté in nonstick pan using Pam or Mazola cooking spray.

[2] About 12 large Roma tomatoes, or use tomatoes of your choice.

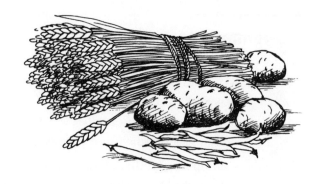

Rice, Grains, Beans, and Potatoes

Fast Chili-Rice Dinner

- 1 lb. ground flank steak or ground turkey
- ⅓ cup chopped onion
- 1 15-oz. can no-salt-added tomato sauce
- ½ cup water
- 1½ teaspoons chili powder
- 2 cloves garlic, minced
- ½ teaspoon ground cumin
- ½ teaspoon dry mustard
- 1 cup diced green pepper
- 1 10-oz. package frozen whole-kernel corn (or 1 cup fresh corn kernels)
- 1 cup cooked brown rice

Brown ground meat and onion in a nonstick skillet. Pour off any fat that accumulates. Add all remaining ingredients except rice. Cover. Bring to a boil, stirring occasionally. Stir in rice and reduce heat. Cover and simmer for 5 minutes. Yields 4 servings.

Plain Brown Rice

Use twice as much water as rice. Bring water to a rolling boil. Add rice and stir with a fork. Bring back to a rolling boil; reduce heat to simmer. Cover and simmer 1 hour. *Do not lift the lid during this time.* Remove from heat; allow rice to sit for 15 minutes. When time is up, remove the lid and fluff the rice with a fork. Rice may be frozen if desired.

Brown Rice Variations

1. Substitute broth for water in cooking. Add a dash of onion and garlic powder.

2. Add sautéed chopped onion, sliced celery, and diced carrots to the liquid when you add the rice.

3. At the end of cooking time, add your favorite herbs or seasonings. You can also add sliced green onions, chopped parsley, diced tomatoes, and diced pimientos. Use your imagination.

Rice Pancakes

1 cup cooked brown rice

4 egg whites, beaten with a fork until frothy

2 tablespoons finely chopped green pepper

2 tablespoons water chestnuts, drained and finely chopped

2 tablespoons finely chopped green onions

2 tablespoons finely chopped celery

Combine all ingredients. Heat a small nonstick skillet, or spray skillet with nonstick cooking spray. Spread rice mixture to cover bottom of the pan. Cook over low heat until bottom of the pancake is slightly brown. Carefully loosen with a spatula, flip over, and slightly cook the other side. Turn onto a warm plate. Good with Foo Yong Sauce (see recipe below). Yields 4 pancakes.

Foo Yong Sauce

Blend 1½ cups chicken stock with 3 tablespoons cornstarch in a small saucepan. Add 1 tablespoon soy sauce. Cook over low heat, stirring constantly, until sauce is thickened. Yields 1½ cups.

Mushroom Rice Pilaf*

½ lb. mushrooms, sliced

½ cup chopped green onions, tops only

2 tablespoons water

2 cups chicken or beef stock, or no-salt-added tomato juice

1 cup uncooked brown rice

Sauté mushrooms and onions in 2 tablespoons water until tender. Add broth and bring to a boil. Place rice in a 2-quart casserole dish and pour the mixture over the rice. Stir. Cover and bake at 350°F. for 1 hour. Yields 6 servings.

Stir-Fried Rice*

3 egg whites

3 tablespoons soy sauce

¼ teaspoon ground ginger

⅛ teaspoon garlic powder

3 tablespoons chicken stock or water

1 cup frozen peas, partially thawed

½ cup sliced mushrooms

3 cups cooked brown rice

¼ cup chopped green onions

Green pepper strips

Carrot strips

Lightly beat egg whites, soy sauce, ginger, and garlic powder. Heat 1 tablespoon of chicken stock or water in a nonstick skillet or wok. Add peas and mushrooms. Stir-fry for 2 minutes. Remove from pan. Add remaining liquid to the pan and heat. Add rice and onions. Stir-fry for 4–6 minutes. Add vegetables and egg mixture. Cook and stir until eggs are set. Garnish with green pepper and carrot strips. Yields 4 servings.

Vegetable Rice Pilaf*

1 cup uncooked brown rice

2 cups chicken broth

1 medium onion, chopped

1 small green pepper, cut into thin strips

1 large tomato, diced

2 tablespoons chopped fresh parsley

Combine the rice, chicken broth, and onion in a 1½-quart saucepan. Bring to a boil. Reduce heat. Cover and simmer for 1 hour. Make sure all of the liquid has been absorbed. Stir in green pepper, tomato, and parsley. Heat through. Yields 6–8 servings.

Bulgur and Brown Rice Pilaf

¼ cup chopped onion

¼ cup chopped celery

½ lb. mushrooms, sliced

1 cup cooked brown rice

⅓ cup bulgur wheat

2 cups + 2 tablespoons chicken or beef broth

Sauté onion, celery, mushrooms, rice, and bulgur in 2 tablespoons broth in a large nonstick skillet. Add 2 cups broth and bring to a boil. Cover and simmer for 30 minutes, or until the grains are tender and broth is absorbed. Yields 8 servings.

Chow Mein Noodles

8 oz. whole-wheat spaghetti, broken in half

Bring 4 quarts water to a racing boil. Slowly add spaghetti and stir once to separate. Boil for 12–15 minutes. Drain and rinse thoroughly with warm water, using a colander. Place spaghetti on a nonstick cookie sheet. Bake at 375°F. for 1 hour, turning noodles often to toast evenly. Yields 8 servings.

Sweet Potatoes in Herb Sauce

1½ lbs. sweet potatoes, peeled and sliced ¼-inch thick

2 tablespoons water

1 cup minced onion

1 clove garlic, crushed

¾ teaspoon crushed dillweed

Dash of white pepper

½ cup plain nonfat yogurt

1 tablespoon lemon juice

2 tablespoons chopped parsley

Steam sweet potatoes about 8–10 minutes or until barely tender. In a nonstick skillet, add 2 tablespoons water, onion, garlic, dillweed, and pepper. Cook until onions are soft. Remove from heat. Stir in the yogurt and lemon juice. Cook over low heat for about 2 minutes. Turn sweet potatoes into a serving dish and toss with sauce. Sprinkle with parsley. Serve immediately. Yields 4–6 servings.

Stir-Fried Vegetables with Brown Rice*

½ lb. broccoli

Juice of 1 lemon

3–4 tablespoons chicken stock

1 medium onion, cut in thin vertical slices, then separated into strips

2 ribs celery, thinly sliced

½ small green pepper, chopped

1 cup fresh or frozen corn kernels, thawed

1 cup fresh or frozen cut green beans, thawed

1 teaspoon crushed oregano

White pepper to taste

2 cups cooked brown rice

Cut flowerets from broccoli stem. Place flowerets in 3 cups water to which lemon juice has been added. Set aside and allow to soak. Peel broccoli stems, then cut into 1-inch slices, then slice again vertically. Heat the chicken stock in a large nonstick skillet over medium heat. Add onion strips, broccoli stem slices, celery, and green pepper. Stir-fry until crisp, about 3 minutes. Drain broccoli flowerets. Add to the onion mixture. Stir in corn, green beans, oregano, and pepper. Stir-fry for 2 minutes or until corn and broccoli flowerets are crispy-tender. Add rice. Stir-fry until hot, about 2 minutes. Yields 4–6 servings.

Cabbage with Lima Beans

    1 cup dried lima beans
3–4 tablespoons chicken broth or water
    1 medium onion, sliced
  ¼ teaspoon caraway seeds
  ½ small head of cabbage, shredded
    3 carrots, sliced
  ½ teaspoon chopped fresh parsley
  ¼ teaspoon summer savory
    2 tablespoons soy sauce
      Dash of white pepper

Soak beans overnight with enough water to cover plus 1 inch more. Do not discard the water. Bring beans to a boil in the soaking water. Reduce heat and simmer for 45 minutes with the lid ajar. Heat chicken broth in a nonstick skillet. Add onion and caraway seeds and sauté for 5 minutes. Add cabbage, carrots, parsley, summer savory, soy sauce, and pepper. Add to the beans. Mix lightly and continue to cook over low heat, covered, for 25 minutes or until cabbage is tender. If necessary, add a little chicken broth or water to keep mixture from sticking to the pan. Yields 4 servings.

Chili

1 lb. red kidney beans
1 16-oz. can unsalted chopped tomatoes
2 fresh skinned and chopped tomatoes
1 6-oz. can tomato paste
3 teaspoons crushed cumin seeds
3 tablespoons chili powder
¼ teaspoon crushed oregano
3 medium chopped onions
2 tablespoons picante sauce (mild or hot)
3 cloves minced garlic
2 tablespoons sherry

Wash beans well and soak overnight in water, enough to allow for the beans to double in bulk. Do not drain. On the following day, bring beans to a boil. Cover and simmer while preparing the other ingredients. Add tomatoes, tomato paste, and cumin seeds and bring to a boil. Lower the heat. Add the remaining ingredients except the sherry. Cover and cook over low heat for 2 hours or until beans are soft, stirring occasionally. Add more water if the mixture becomes too thick. Add sherry just before removing from the heat. Adjust seasoning to your liking. Yields 6–8 servings.

Steamed Oriental Vegetables and Brown Rice*

1¾ cups sliced fresh mushrooms
1½ cups thinly sliced Chinese cabbage
1½ cups diagonally sliced celery
3 carrots, cut into matchsticks
2 large onions, thinly sliced

1 large green pepper, thinly sliced
1 8-oz. can water chestnuts, drained and sliced
½ cup sliced bamboo shoots
¼ cup chicken broth
¾ cup fresh snow peas
3 cups beans sprouts
1 8-oz. can unsweetened pineapple chunks

Combine all vegetables except snow peas and bean sprouts in a large steamer or wok. Add the chicken broth. Cover and steam for 4–5 minutes. Add snow peas, bean sprouts, and pineapple. Continue cooking for about 3–4 minutes. Mix thoroughly. If desired, sprinkle with low-sodium soy sauce diluted with equal amount of water. Serve over hot brown rice or Chow Mein Noodles (see page 232). Yields 6–8 servings.

Stuffed Baked Potatoes*

4 medium baking potatoes
1 cup dry-curd or nonfat cottage cheese
¼ cup plain nonfat yogurt
1 tablespoon nonfat milk (or more for desired consistency)
½ cup finely chopped onion
2 tablespoons water
⅛ teaspoon white pepper
Chopped chives

Bake well-scrubbed potatoes in a 450°F. oven for 1 hour. Mash the cottage cheese with yogurt and milk. Mix well. Sauté onion in 2 tablespoons water in a nonstick skillet until tender. Cut a thin slice off the top of each potato. Remove the pulp and save the shell. Combine cottage cheese mixture with pepper, onion, and potato pulp. Mash. Stuff the potato mixture into the shells. Reheat the potatoes in a 350°F. oven until hot. Sprinkle with chopped chives before serving. Yields 4 servings.

Oven French Fries*

2 large potatotes
2 egg whites, beaten
   Dillweed, crushed

Preheat oven to 425°F. Peel and cut potatoes into wedges. Dip the wedges into beaten egg whites and sprinkle with dill. Bake on a nonstick pan at 425°F. for 25–30 minutes. Yields 2 servings.

Karen's Crusty Broiler-Fried Potatoes*

Bake 1 potato in microwave for 10 minutes (or in conventional oven for 1 hour at 450°F.). Cool and slice as thinly as possible. Line broiler with foil. Crush one garlic clove and brush garlic across foil (optional). Spray foil lightly with Pam or Mazola nonstick cooking spray. Broil potato slices on high for 5–7 minutes a side. Delicious! Yields 1 serving.

Scalloped Potatoes

6 cups sliced potatoes
1½ cups nonfat skim milk
1 clove garlic, crushed
1 large onion, minced

1 teaspoon dillweed

⅛ teaspoon white pepper

2 tablespoons potato starch or cornstarch combined with 3 tablespoons water to make a thin paste

Mazola or Pam nonstick cooking spray

½ cup plain nonfat yogurt

2 teaspoons chopped parsley

4 tablespoons chopped green onions

Preheat oven to 350°F. Place sliced potatoes in bowl of cold water to cover. Set aside. Bring milk to a boil. Add garlic, onion, dillweed, and white pepper. Add potato starch or cornstarch mixed with water. Stir to keep from lumping. Drain potatoes and spread in a glass baking dish sprayed with cooking spray. Pour milk mixture over potatoes. Top with yogurt. Cover with foil. Bake in 350°F. oven for 30 minutes. Remove foil and allow to bake 30 minutes longer. Garnish with parsley and green onions. Yields 4 servings.

Spicy Lima Beans

1 10-oz. package frozen lima beans (or 1 cup fresh limas)

2 tablespoons Tomato Ketchup (see page 226) or tomato sauce

1 teaspoon minced onion

Dash of white pepper

Cook lima beans in small amount of water according to package directions (cover fresh limas with water and cook until tender). Add ketchup, onion, and pepper. Stir gently over low heat for a few minutes until the liquid is almost absorbed. Yields 2 servings.

Corn Oriental

½ cup chicken broth
½ cup chopped green onions, including part of the tops
1½ cups sliced mushrooms
1 10-oz. package frozen pea pods, thawed
1 8-oz. can water chestnuts, drained, sliced, and peeled
3 cups cooked corn kernels
1 teaspoon soy sauce diluted with 1 teaspoon water

In a wok or nonstick skillet, heat chicken broth. Add remaining ingredients and cook over low heat, stirring, until vegetables are barely tender and heated through (about 5 minutes). Yields 6–8 servings.

Corn on the Cob*

Basic for any amount of servings. To steam: Steam corn for 5 minutes in a steamer. To boil: Bring water to a rolling boil and carefully drop the corn into the pot. Let the water return to a full boil. Cook for 5–7 minutes. Serve with lemon wedges or plain.

Kidney Beans with Garlic Sauce

1 cup dried kidney beans
4 cups cold water
1 rib celery
1 carrot
3 tablespoons apple juice concentrate
2 bay leaves
Dash of white pepper
Chopped parsley

Soak beans in water overnight. Discard soaking water. Put beans in a kettle with 4 cups cold water, celery, carrot, apple juice concentrate, and bay leaves. Bring to a boil. Turn heat down and simmer uncovered for about 1 hour or until beans are tender. Remove carrot, celery, and bay leaves. Add pepper. Simmer until there is almost no liquid left. Serve hot or cold with Garlic Sauce (see below). Garnish with parsley. Yields 6–8 servings.

Garlic Sauce

4 medium potatoes, peeled and quartered
4½ cups water
6 cloves garlic
4 tablespoons apple cider vinegar

Boil potatoes in 4½ cups water until barely tender. Place ½ cup of the potato water in a blender. Add garlic and potatoes; blend. Add vinegar a little at a time and blend until smooth. Chill before serving. Yields 2 cups.

Meatballs

1 lb. ground flank steak or ground turkey
½ cup dry sourdough bread crumbs, or enough matzo meal to bind the mixture
2 egg whites, slightly beaten
1 tablespoon minced onion
½ teaspoon chili powder

Combine all ingredients and mix well. Shape into meatballs. Arrange meatballs on a nonstick pan and bake at 450°F. for 10 minutes. See below for cooking meatballs in sauce.

Sauce for Spaghetti and Meatballs

¾ cup chopped onions
½ teaspoon minced garlic
2 16-oz. cans unsalted tomatoes
1 6-oz. can tomato paste
1½ cups water
½ cup dry sherry (optional)
4 tablespoons apple juice concentrate, thawed
1 tablespoon apple cider vinegar
1 bay leaf
½ teaspoon oregano leaves
½ teaspoon basil leaves
⅛ teaspoon ground cloves

Sauté onions and garlic in a nonstick pan with a small amount of water until soft. Add tomatoes, tomato paste, water, sherry, apple juice concentrate, vinegar, and seasonings. Simmer uncovered for 30 minutes, stirring occasionally. Cover and simmer 30 minutes more. Add meatballs to sauce. Cover and simmer 15 minutes. Stir to cover meatballs with sauce. Remove bay leaf before serving. Serve with whole-wheat spaghetti or wheat-free corn pasta or thin spaghetti. Yields 6 servings.

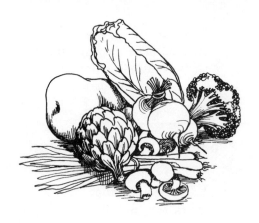

Vegetables

Hints for Serving Vegetables and Fruits

Wash, pare, cut or shred vegetables just before cooking. Soaking vegetables in water drains out the water-soluble vitamins and minerals.

Steam fresh vegetables or boil quickly in a small amount of water in a tightly covered pan. Cook only until crispy-tender.

Fresh or frozen vegetables provide the necessary vitamins and minerals needed for a well-balanced meal. There is a wide variety available. Wash all fresh fruits and vegetables before cooking and eating to remove pesticides.

Prepare vegetable salads just before serving to retain vitamins.

For innovative and tasty salads, learn to recognize salad greens and mix different types together.

Bibb lettuce. Deep green, leaves are sweet and tender.

Boston lettuce. Velvety leaves that are tender and succulent.

Curly endive. Feathered leaves, rather bitter flavor; adds interest to mixed green salads.

Chives. Slim buds and delicate tops. Snip finely and scatter in any salad for a refined onion flavor.

Escarole. Dark green leaves edged in yellow; slightly sharp flavor. Excellent in mixed green salads.

Iceberg lettuce. Compact head, brittle leaves. Tear to use in tossed salads or cut into quarters to use alone.

Romaine lettuce. Cylindrical head, spoon-shaped leaves. It has a pleasant sweet flavor.

Scallions. Tender young onions with a vigorous flavor.

Spinach. Deep green color, lively flavor.

Watercress. Dark green and lacy. Sharp peppery flavor, good for garnish.

Broccoli and Rice

2 cups + 2 tablespoons chicken broth
1 cup uncooked brown rice
1 medium onion, chopped
1 clove garlic, minced
1 10-oz. package frozen chopped broccoli, thawed

Bring 2 cups chicken broth to a boil. Add rice. Reduce heat, cover, and cook for 1 hour. Sauté onion and garlic in 2 tablespoons chicken broth until tender. Stir onion, garlic, and broccoli into the rice. Cover and continue to cook until all of the liquid has been absorbed (about 5 minutes). Yields 6 servings.

Dilled Carrots in Wine Sauce

8 medium carrots, cut into coins
½ cup + 2 tablespoons water
½ cup dry white wine (optional)

    1 tablespoon fresh lemon juice
    1 tablespoon minced onion
    ¼ teaspoon garlic powder
    ½ teaspoon dillweed
    2 tablespoons cornstarch

Place carrots in a saucepan. Add ½ cup water, wine, lemon juice, onion, garlic powder, and dillweed. Cover and cook until tender-crisp. Dissolve cornstarch in 2 tablespoons water. Stir into carrot mixture. Cook and stir until thickened. Yields 6 servings.

Steamed Chayote

    1 medium chayote, scrubbed well
    1 medium onion, chopped
    1 clove garlic, crushed
    3 tablespoons low-sodium V8 juice or water
    1 large tomato, chopped
    ¼ teaspoon diced mild chili pepper
    ¼ teaspoon oregano
    2 tablespoons chopped parsley

If the skin is tender, you can cook a chayote without peeling. Slice the chayote right through the seed to make slices ⅛-inch thick. Cut the slices in half. This makes about 3 cups. Set aside. In a nonstick skillet, sauté onion and garlic in V8 juice or water over medium heat until soft. Add the chayote, tomato, chili pepper, and oregano. Stir. Cover tightly and cook for 10–15 minutes or until chayote is just barely tender and the liquid is absorbed. Stir in the parsley. Turn into a serving dish and serve at once. Yields 3–4 servings.

Basic Cooking Instructions for Butternut Squash

To bake whole: Wash, dry, and place squash in a baking dish. Bake at 375°F. in a small amount of water for 1 hour, or until skin can be pierced easily with a fork.

To steam: Peel, seed, and cut squash into 1-inch rings or chunks. Steam for 20 minutes or until tender. Try seasoning with cinnamon, nutmeg, and cloves.

Butternut Squash Casserole

1 medium-size butternut squash (or any other winter squash, such as pumpkin or banana squash)

3 egg whites, beaten lightly

¼ cup nonfat skim milk

1 teaspoon ground nutmeg

Peel squash, slice in half lengthwise, and remove the seeds. Cut into 1-inch slices in a saucepan. Cover with water. Cover and cook until tender, about 10 minutes. Drain off water; mash squash. Combine with other ingredients and mix well. Pour into a baking dish. Bake at 375°F. for 40–50 minutes. Yields 4–6 servings.

Basic Cooking Instructions for Spaghetti Squash

This is an easy and fun squash to prepare; it reheats well and freezes well.

To prepare whole squash: Boil for 45 minutes or steam for 35 minutes. Test with a fork before removing from heat. To bake, place on a baking sheet and pierce with a sharp fork before baking. Bake at 350°F. for 1½ hours.

To bake halved squash: Cut squash lengthwise and remove the seeds. Place squash in a baking dish, cut side down, and add a small amount of water. Bake at 350°F. for 45 minutes or until tender. Remove from oven. Run a fork over the inside of the cooked squash to fluff up the pastalike strands. May be served in the shell with tomato sauce or spaghetti sauce. Also good chilled and used in salads. To remove the squash from the shells, scoop out the insides carefully with two forks and fluff together with whatever mixture you have prepared.

Spaghetti Squash Stir-Fry

3   green onions, finely sliced
3   celery ribs, finely sliced
3   tablespoons chicken broth
1   medium spaghetti squash, cooked (see Basic Cooking Instructions above)
2   tablespoons soy sauce
1   tablespoon dry sherry

In a nonstick skillet, sauté the green onions and celery in chicken broth for 3 minutes over medium heat. Add the spaghetti squash, soy sauce, and sherry. Stir-fry until completely heated. Yields 6–8 servings.

Pasta Pretender

1   lb. ground flank steak or ground turkey
1   medium onion, chopped
1   16-oz. can unsalted tomatoes, cut up

2 tablespoons juice from the tomatoes

1 teaspoon crushed dried basil leaves

½ teaspoon crushed oregano

Cooked spaghetti squash (see Basic Cooking Instructions above)

1 teaspoon grated sapsago, Parmesan, or Romano cheese

In a nonstick skillet, sauté the meat and onion in 2 tablespoons of juice from the tomatoes. Add tomatoes, basil, and oregano. Simmer until most of the juices evaporate. Pour the meat sauce over cooked spaghetti squash. Sprinkle grated cheese on top. Serve in the spaghetti squash shells. Yields 4–6 servings.

Stir-Fry Veggies*

3 tablespoons chicken broth

3 ribs celery, finely sliced

2 carrots, cut into matchsticks

1 lb. broccoli, cut in flowerets with stems peeled and sliced

1 cup sliced mushrooms

Any other seasonal vegetable desired

1 teaspoon grated lemon rind

1 clove garlic, mashed in garlic press

½ teaspoon ground ginger

In a large nonstick skillet, heat chicken broth over medium heat. Add all remaining ingredients. Stir-fry for 5–6 minutes or until vegetables are tender. Yields 4–6 servings.

Yam Pineapple Bake

     5 unpeeled yams or sweet potatoes, well scrubbed
    ½ cup crushed pineapple, packed in its own juice (no
       sugar added)
    ½ teaspoon cinnamon
    ¼ teaspoon nutmeg
     1 egg white, stiffly beaten
     1 teaspoon grated orange rind (optional)
       Pam or Mazola nonstick cooking spray
     2 tablespoons kirsch or your favorite brandy

Cook yams in 2 quarts boiling water, covered, for 20–
30 minutes. Drain. When cool enough to handle, peel
and mash yams. Add the pineapple and its juice, cinnamon, and nutmeg. Mix well. Fold in stiffly beaten
egg white. Add grated orange rind. Turn into a nonstick baking pan sprayed with cooking spray. Sprinkle
kirsch over mixture. Bake uncovered in a 350°F. oven
for 15–20 minutes. Yields 6–8 servings.

Zucchini Italiano*

     3 tablespoons chicken broth
     2 medium onions, sliced into rings
     2 cloves garlic, minced
     1 teaspoon crushed oregano leaves
    ¼ teaspoon crushed basil leaves
     1 6-oz. can tomato paste
    ¼ cup water
     2 lbs. zucchini, cut into ½-inch slices

In a nonstick skillet, combine chicken broth, onions,
garlic, oregano, and basil. Cook until onions are tender.

Add tomato paste, water, and zucchini. Cover and cook over low heat for 20 minutes, stirring occasionally. Yields 6–8 servings.

Yellow Squash and Carrot Dish

1 lb. yellow squash
1 medium onion, grated
3 carrots, grated
2 teaspoons chopped parsley
3 ribs celery, cut into medium diagonal slices
1½ teaspoons dillweed
⅔ cups oat or rice flour[1]
2 tablespoons potato starch or cornstarch
½ teaspoon low-sodium baking powder
2 egg whites beaten to soft-peak stage
Nonstick cooking spray
1 shredded wheat biscuit, crushed

Steam squash until soft enough to mash. Cool. Preheat oven to 350°F. Mash squash and add onion, carrots, parsley, celery, and dillweed. Mix together. Combine flour, potato starch, and baking powder. Add to squash mixture and mix well. Fold in stiffly beaten egg whites. Pour into a nonstick pan sprayed with cooking spray. Top with crushed Shredded Wheat. Bake in a preheated 350°F. oven for 45–50 minutes. Yields 6 generous servings.

Use recipe for Oat Flour below or purchase rice flour at health-food store.

Oat Flour

In a blender or food processor, process 1½ cups rolled oats for 1 minute or until completely ground. Yields 1 cup flour.

Green Beans and Mushrooms*

1½ cups sliced mushrooms
 2 tablespoons water
 2 teaspoons dry sherry
 ⅛ teaspoon ground nutmeg
 ¼ teaspoon ground majoram
 1 10-oz. package frozen cut green beans, or ¾ lb. fresh green beans
   Cherry tomatoes, cut in halves

Place the mushrooms in a medium-size nonstick skillet with 2 tablespoons water. Cook 2–3 minutes. Stir in sherry, nutmeg, and marjoram. Add green beans and simmer, covered, for 10 minutes. Garnish with cherry tomatoes. Yields 4 servings.

Stuffed Pattypan Squash*

6–10 pattypan squash (light-green summer squash)
   1 10-oz. package frozen mixed vegetables

Steam squash until tender. While squash is steaming, cook mixed vegetables according to package directions. Scoop out cooked squash, leaving a shell about ½ inch thick. Combine squash pulp with drained vegetables. Fill squash shell with vegetable mixture. Yields 6 servings.

Stir-Fry Broccoli*

1½ lbs. fresh broccoli, cut in flowerets with stems peeled and sliced thinly
 4 carrots, cut into matchsticks
 1 cup sliced mushrooms
 ¼ cup sliced onion
 2 tablespoons water
 1 cup fresh bean sprouts
 2 teaspoons cornstarch
 1 cup chicken broth
 1 clove garlic, minced
 ¼ teaspoon ground ginger
   Scant ⅛ teaspoon white pepper
 1 red pepper, cut into strips

In a large nonstick skillet, combine broccoli, carrots, mushrooms, onion, and 2 tablespoons water. Stir-fry over medium heat for about 3–4 minutes. Add bean sprouts. Stir cornstarch into a little cold water in a measuring cup. Add enough chicken broth to make 1 cup. Add to vegetable mixture along with garlic, ginger, and white pepper. Simmer about 3 minutes, stirring, until liquid thickens and vegetables are tender-crisp. Garnish with red pepper strips. Yields 4 servings.

Ratatouille*

 3 medium onions, thinly sliced
 2 tablespoons chicken stock, no-salt-added tomato juice, or water
 1 medium eggplant, peeled and cubed
 3 large tomatoes, peeled and cut up

3 or 4 zucchini, cubed
   3 green peppers, cut in small strips
   ½ lb. mushrooms, sliced
   1 6-oz. can tomato paste
   2 cloves garlic, mashed
   1 teaspoon Italian seasoning
   ½ teaspoon dillweed
   ½ teaspoon oregano
   ¼ teaspoon white pepper
   1 bay leaf
   ¼ teaspoon grated lemon rind
   1 tablespoon Angostura bitters (optional)

In a large nonstick skillet, sauté onions in chicken stock, water, or tomato juice until translucent. Add remaining ingredients while stirring lightly. Place in baking dish. Cover loosely with foil and bake in 350°F. oven for 40 minutes. (Some of the liquid will evaporate.) Remove bay leaf. Yields 4 servings.

Aubergine a l'Indochinoise

Pam or Mazola nonstick cooking spray
   4 medium eggplant, cut in ½-inch slices
   4 cups Marinara Sauce (see pages 46 and 227)
   3 cups cooked brown rice
   ¼ cup grated sapsago cheese
   ¼ cup crushed shredded wheat

In a nonstick baking pan sprayed with nonstick cooking spray, layer eggplant, Marinara Sauce, and rice, using sauce for every other layer. Finish with eggplant. Top with grated cheese and crushed shredded wheat. Bake at 350°F. for 45 minutes. Yield 8 servings.

Squash Souffle*

2 cups cooked millet (cook according to directions on package)

1 large banana squash, peeled[1]

2 carrots, peeled[1]

½ clove garlic

1 teaspoon fresh lemon juice

½ teaspoon cinnamon

¼ teaspoon white pepper

4 egg whites

Pam or Mazola nonstick cooking spray

Steam the squash and carrots for 20 minutes. Preheat oven to 325°F.

Place the vegetables in a blender. Add garlic, lemon juice, cinnamon, and pepper. Blend until smooth.

In a separate bowl, beat the egg whites until stiff peaks form. Gently fold in the squash mixture. Spray an 11 × 14 × 2-inch nonstick baking pan with cooking spray. Place the cooked millet in the bottom of the pan. Pour the squash mixture over the millet. Bake in a 325°F. oven for 20–25 minutes. Yields 6 servings as an entrée or 8 as a side dish.

[1] *Variation:* Substitute broccoli, asparagus, or other green vegetables of your choice.

Pasta Primavera*

1 cone sapsago cheese[1]

4 medium-size carrots, cut in 1-inch pieces

[1] Sapsago is a hard, nonfat cheese that comes in the shape of a small cone. If unavailable, use a *very small* amount of Romano or Parmesan cheese.

1 lb. broccoli, cut into bite-size pieces

2 medium zucchini, cut in 1-inch pieces

½ lb. spaghetti or corn pasta

1 cup chicken broth

3 teaspoons potato starch or cornstarch

2 cloves garlic, minced

1 lb. cherry tomatoes, halved

2 tablespoons water

1 teaspoon crushed basil

½ lb. mushrooms, sliced

1 10-oz. package frozen peas, slightly thawed

¾ cup chopped parsley

Grate sapsago cheese in a food processor and set aside.

Steam carrots, broccoli, and zucchini until crispy-tender. Put in a large bowl and set aside.

Cook spaghetti al dente. Drain and set aside.

Combine chicken broth and potato starch or cornstarch. Stir until smooth. Bring to a boil, then reduce heat to simmer. Cook and stir until thickened. Set aside.

Sauté garlic and tomatoes in a large nonstick skillet with 2 tablespoons water for 2 minutes. Stir in basil and mushrooms. Cook 2 more minutes. Stir in peas and parsley. Cook 1 more minute. Add to steamed vegetables in the bowl.

In the large nonstick skillet, add spaghetti to the thickened chicken broth mixture and toss to coat. Stir in the vegetables. Heat slowly until hot. Sprinkle the cheese lightly over the Pasta Primavera. Yields 6 servings.

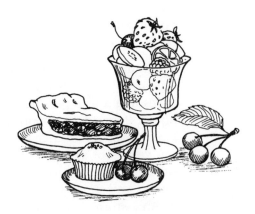

Desserts

Yogurt*

- 1 quart nonfat skim milk
- 2 acidophilus capsules (available in the health-food section of your supermarket, or in health-food stores), **or**
- 1 cup plain low-fat yogurt

Scald the milk (do not boil). Add powder from the capsules, or add yogurt.[1] Let sit in a warm spot in your kitchen overnight. Store in the refrigerator. To make your next batch of yogurt, add a cup of this yogurt to a quart of scalded skim milk. Use the same procedure each time.

[1] The yogurt as well as the capsules are a source of live acidophilus bacteria, which will convert the milk to yogurt.

Orange Delight

- ⅓ cup raisins
- 4 oranges, peeled and sliced
- 3 tablespoons kirsch (wild-cherry liqueur)

1 cup fresh cranberries
Dash of Angostura bitters

To plump raisins, pour enough boiling water over the raisins to cover them. Set aside. Arrange the orange slices in a round pie dish. Drain the raisins, saving the liquid. Pour 3 tablespoons of the raisin liquid and the kirsch over the oranges. Cover the dish with foil and refrigerate for several hours. Pour off the liquid into a saucepan and bring to a boil. Add cranberries and raisins and simmer for about 3–4 minutes. Add a dash of Angostura. Pour the sauce over the oranges and chill. Yields 4 servings.

Apple Pie

Grape Nuts pie crust (see below)
2 large baking apples, thinly sliced (about 2 cups)
6 tablespoons water, divided
1 tablespoon unflavored gelatin
¼ cup boiling water
1 cup unsweetened applesauce
¼ cup apple juice concentrate, thawed
1 teaspoon apple pie spice
¼ teaspoon cardamom
½ teaspoon Angostura bitters
Mock Whipping Kream (optional, see page 257)

Prepare pie crust and set aside. Combine apples in a saucepan with ¼ cup water. Bring to a boil, cover, and cook 3–4 minutes. Soften gelatin in 2 tablespoons cold water. Add ¼ cup boiling water to gelatin and stir until completely dissolved. Combine gelatin with apple-sauce, cooked apples, apple juice concentrate, spices, and Angostura. Cool. Spoon mixture into the crust and refrigerate for at least 2 hours. If desired, top each slice with 1 teaspoon Mock Whipping Kream. Yields an 8-inch pie.

Grape-Nuts Crust

1 cup Grape Nuts cereal

½ cup cooked wheat berries (whole-grain wheat cereal)

½ teaspoon vanilla extract

Combine ingredients; mix well. Line sides and bottom of 8-inch pie pan with mixture.

Mock Whipping Kream

Pour evaporated skim milk into ice tray; place in freezer until ice crystals form around the edge. In a chilled bowl, beat the milk into a peak. Use immediately. To freeze: Drop by teaspoonfuls on a cookie sheet and freeze. When completely firm, place in an airtight bag. Remove only the amount you need about 5 minutes before serving.

Fruit Juice Whip #1

1¼ cups water, divided

1 envelope unflavored gelatin

1 6-oz. can frozen concentrated fruit juice of your choice (do not use frozen pineapple juice)

2 egg whites

Add ½ cup water to the gelatin. Place in a small sauce-pan over low heat and stir constantly until gelatin is dissolved. Remove from heat and stir in remaining ¾ cup water and frozen juice. Stir until juice is melted. Chill until slightly thicker than unbeaten egg whites. Add egg whites and beat with electric mixer until mixture begins to hold its shape. Spoon into sherbet dishes. Chill until firm. Yields 8 servings.

Fruit Juice Whip #2

½ cup water

1 envelope unflavored gelatin

1 6-oz. can fruit juice concentrate (apple, orange, grape-fruit, or cranberry)

2¼ cups low-fat buttermilk

Add water to gelatin and place over low heat, stirring constantly until gelatin is dissolved. Empty fruit juice concentrate into a bowl and add buttermilk. Stir gelatin into buttermilk mixture. Pour into an ice tray and place in freezer. When partially frozen, remove mixture to a bowl and beat until smooth. Return to tray and freeze until firm. Yields 8 servings.

Fruit Medley*

1 apple, cut into bite-size pieces

2 oranges, peeled and sliced

2 bananas, peeled and sliced

2 ripe pears (Bosc, Comice, or Anjou), cut into bite-size pieces

1 cup black or purple grapes, seeded and halved

½ cup dry white wine (optional)[1]

½ cup fresh-squeezed orange juice (remove seeds, do not strain)

Combine fruit and toss lightly. Combine orange juice and wine. Pour over fruit and mix gently to coat the fruit. Chill at least 2 hours. Yields 6–8 servings.

[1] Do not use the wine on fruit day.

Spiced Vanilla Sherbet

½ cup evaporated skim milk

1 tablespoon lemon juice

½ teaspoon vanilla extract

¼ teaspoon nutmeg or cinnamon

Combine ingredients and pour into an ice tray. Freeze only until ice crystals form. Chill bowl and beaters of electric mixer. Remove sherbet from tray and whip with mixer until firm. Pour back into ice tray and freeze until firm. Yields 1 pint.

Easy Peach Dessert

4 large peaches

¾ cup dry red wine

¼ cup apple juice concentrate

Peel and pit the peaches, cut into bite-size pieces, and place in a bowl. Pour wine and apple juice concentrate over the peaches. Chill in the refrigerator for at least 1 hour. If desired, drop a dollop of Angostura Yogurt Sauce (see page 225) over each serving. Yields 4–6 servings.

Nectarine Sherbet

1 envelope unflavored gelatin
¼ cup apple juice concentrate
1 cup nonfat skim milk
2 tablespoons lemon juice
6 large nectarines, peeled and sliced
1 egg white

Soften gelatin in apple juice concentrate. Place over low heat and stir until gelatin is completely dissolved. Combine milk and lemon juice with dissolved gelatin. Puree nectarines in blender and add to gelatin mixture. Pour into 1 large or 2 small ice trays and freeze until almost firm. Chill mixer bowl and beaters. Add egg white to gelatin mixture and beat with electric beater until fluffy. Return to ice tray and freeze until firm. Remove from freezer a few minutes before serving to soften slightly. Yields about 3 pints.

Fresh Fruit Perrier Sparkle

1 cup Perrier mineral water
1 6-oz. can apple juice concentrate, thawed
1 6-oz. can orange juice concentrate, thawed
1 medium pineapple, cut into cubes
1 pint strawberries, cleaned and quartered
Mint sprigs

Combine Perrier, apple juice concentrate, and orange juice concentrate in blender or food processor. Blend at high speed for a few seconds. Pour into ice trays and freeze just until ice crystals form (not frozen solid). Spoon fruit into dessert dishes. Top with juice mixture and garnish with mint sprigs. Yields 12 servings.

Frozen Apple Mousse

1 13-oz. can evaporated skim milk, chilled overnight
1 tablespoon lime juice
1 6-oz. can frozen apple juice concentrate (do not thaw)
1 tablespoon Angostura bitters
½ teaspoon nutmeg or cinnamon
3 tablespoon Kirsch or gin
½ teaspoon grated lemon rind
½ teaspoon grated orange rind

Chill mixer bowl and beaters. Combine milk and lime juice and beat rapidly until stiff. (Placing the bowl in a pan of ice cubes while you are beating the mixture helps to make the mousse stiff.) Add remaining ingredients and continue beating until mixed. Pour mixture into a well-chilled shallow 11 × 13-inch baking pan and freeze for 4–6 hours. Yields 12 servings.

Roasted Chestnuts

Rinse chestnuts, do not dry. Cut an X on the flat side of the shell. Put chestnuts in a cast-iron frying pan on the range. Cover the pan with a Pyrex bowl. Turn flame on medium heat for 5 minutes. Turn down to low for 10 minutes. Turn chestnuts over and roast for 10 minutes more. When cool enough to handle, peel and eat. Enjoy!

Le Frozen Banana Whip

6 very ripe bananas, sliced
2 tablespoons plain nonfat yogurt
1 tablespoon brandy

¼ teaspoon Angostura bitters (optional)

1 teaspoon grated orange or lemon peel

Freeze bananas on a nonstick pan. When bananas are frozen hard, put them in a food processor and blend with yogurt, brandy, and Angostura until smooth. Spoon the mixture into sherbet dishes and sprinkle with grated citrus peel. Return to freezer until very firm. Allow to stand at room temperature for 10 minutes before serving. Yields 8–10 servings.

Fruited Rice

¼ cup plain nonfat yogurt

2 cups cooked brown rice, chilled

2 cups fresh fruit and berries in season

Stir yogurt into chilled rice. Fold in the fruit mixture. Yields 8 servings.

Fruit Compote*

1 large banana, sliced

1 cup plain nonfat yogurt

1 cup fresh pineapple, diced

1 cup melon of your choice, diced

6 large strawberries with stems left on

Place banana and yogurt in blender and blend until smooth. Put equal amounts of pineapple and melon in dessert cups and spoon the banana-yogurt mixture over the fruit. Garnish each serving with a strawberry. Yields 6 generous servings.

Fruit Punch

    1 6-oz. can apple juice concentrate, thawed
 1½ cups water, divided
    2 cups fresh pineapple wedges
    5 medium bananas
    1 cup fresh-squeezed orange juice
  ½ cup fresh lemon juice
      Grenadine for color (optional)
      Ice cubes
    4 thin slices of orange

> Combine apple juice concentrate and 1 cup water.
> Bring to a boil. Set aside to cool. In a blender, combine
> half the pineapple and ¼ cup water. Blend for 1 min-
> ute. Repeat using the remaining pineapple and ¼ cup
> water. Pour into a pitcher or large bowl. Peel and slice
> 3 bananas and place half the slices in the blender.
> Blend for 1 minute. Repeat using remaining banana
> slices. Add to the pineapple mixture along with apple
> juice concentrate, orange juice, and lemon juice. Add
> enough grenadine to give desired pink color. Peel re-
> maining 2 bananas. Cut them in half lengthwise and
> place each half in a tall glass. Fill with ice cubes. Pour
> the punch into the glasses. Float a thin slice of orange
> on top of each glass. Yields 4 servings, about 1½ quarts.

No-Cooking Applesauce*

    1 tablespoon fresh lemon juice
  ⅛ teaspoon cardamom
  ⅛ teaspoon ground cinnamon
    4 medium-large apples, peeled, cored, and quartered

In blender or food processor, place lemon juice, cardamom, cinnamon, and half of the apples. Blend until mixture looks like applesauce. Gradually add the remaining apples and blend until smooth. Yields 2½–3 cups.

Fruit Juice Ice

   1 envelope unflavored gelatin
3¼ cups + 2 tablespoons water, divided
   1 6-oz. can apple juice concentrate, thawed
   2 cups fresh-squeezed orange juice
  ¼ cup lime juice
  ¼ cup kirsch (wild-cherry liqueur)
      Peel of 1 lemon, grated finely
      Peel of 1 orange, grated finely

Soften gelatin in ¼ cup water. Set aside. Bring apple juice concentrate and 3 cups + 2 tablespoons water to a boil (4 cups of liquid total). Boil for 2 minutes. Remove from heat. Stir in softened gelatin until dissolved. Pour into a large bowl and let sit for a few minutes. Stir in remaining ingredients. When completely cool, pour into a large pan and freeze until firm. Thaw slightly. Chill mixer bowl and beaters. Beat mixture until fluffy. Return to pan, cover with foil, and freeze. Yields about 8 servings.

Kiwi Fruit Drink

   1 kiwi, peeled and sliced
  ½ cup fresh-squeezed orange juice
   1 banana, peeled and sliced

Crushed ice

Mint sprigs

Combine kiwi, orange juice, and banana in blender and blend until frothy. Serve in tall glasses over crushed ice. Garnish with mint sprigs. Yields 2 servings.

Melon Garni*

1 cantaloupe

1 tablespoon lemon juice

1 cup seedless grapes

1 cup watermelon balls

Other fruit, such as strawberries, cherries, or other types of melon may be substituted

Cut cantaloupe in half, preserving a one-inch-wide strip connected at each side to serve as the handle of a basket-shaped shell formed by the rind. Scoop out the flesh of the cantaloupe, maintaining the basket shape. Coat the inside of the cantaloupe with lemon juice, saving any extra. Combine fruit in the shell. Pour any remaining lemon juice over the mixture. Chill until ready to serve. Yields 6 servings.

Noodle Kugel

1 lb. dry-curd or low-fat cottage cheese, hoop cheese, or nonfat ricotta

½ cup nonfat skim milk

2 egg whites

2 teaspoons vanilla extract

2 medium-sized Red or Golden Delicious apples, peeled and chopped

½ cup raisins

1 teaspoon cinnamon

1 10-oz. package corn pasta, whole-wheat noodles, or regular noodles, cooked and drained

Pam or Mazola nonstick cooking spray (optional)

In a food processor, combine the cheese and milk. Process until blended. Add egg whites and vanilla. Blend. Combine apples, raisins, and cinnamon and stir into the cheese mixture. Combine all ingredients with noodles. Pour into an 8 × 12-inch glass baking dish sprayed with nonstick cooking spray, or a nonstick baking pan. Sprinkle additional cinnamon on top. Bake at 350°F. for 30 minutes. Yields 6–8 servings.

Christi's Basic Muffin Recipe*

1½ cups whole-wheat flour

⅓ cup oat bran

⅓ cup wheat bran

3 tablespoons nonfat dry milk powder

2 teaspoons Rumsford baking powder[1]

½ teaspoon freshly grated orange peel

2 teaspoons cinnamon

5 egg whites

5 tablespoons honey

3 tablespoons oil (canola, olive, or safflower)

2 teaspoons vanilla extract (don't use imitation vanilla flavoring)

---

[1] Rumsford baking powder is lower in sodium than other brands and contains no aluminum sulfate.

Variations (choose one):

1 cup shredded carrots

1 cup shredded zucchini

1 cup mashed bananas

1 cup chopped berries or cherries

1 cup blueberries, fresh or frozen

Preheat oven to 350°F. Stir together the first seven ingredients in a large bowl. Puree remaining ingredients in blender or use hand mixer (this is a very important step). Add pureed liquid to dry mixture and stir well (DO NOT BEAT). The mixture will be thick like a cookie dough. Mix in choice of variation until well distributed. By hand, divide the dough into 12 portions and put into paper-lined muffin cups. Bake at 350°F. for about 17 minutes, or until top begins to darken and center springs back when lightly pressed. Yields 12 muffins.

Index of Recipes